All is Well

The Art {and Science} of Personal Well-Being

All is Well

The Art {and Science} of Personal Well-Being

Marilynn Preston

Creators Publishing
Hermosa Beach, CA

The enso contains the perfect and imperfect;
that is why it's always complete.
—Kazuaki Tanahashi

All is Well
The Art {and Science} of Personal Well-Being

Cover design by Peggy Pfeiffer
Cover art courtesy of Kazuaki Tanahashi
Back cover author photo by Ellen Warner
Winter, Spring, Summer, Autumn photos by Barbara Bonfigli
Creative Coordinator Peter Kaminski

CREATORS PUBLISHING
737 3rd St
Hermosa Beach, CA 90254
  A Blue-Zone Community
310-337-7003

Library of Congress Control Number: 2017931018
ISBN (print): 9781945630439
ISBN (ebook): 9781945630446

First Edition
Printed in the United States of America
1 3 5 7 9 10 8 6 4 2

In gratitude to my readers. Without you, nothing.

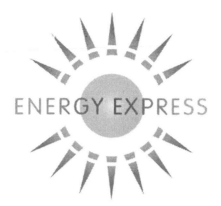

Tell me, what is it you plan to do
with your one wild and precious life?
—Mary Oliver

Table of Contents

Winter

Spring

Summer

Autumn

Introduction

It was 1972, in Chicago, and my husband and I made a bold and crazy decision to take our 10-speed bicycles to France and ride through the gorgeous vineyards of Bordeaux and Burgundy. We had no idea what we were getting into.

I decided I'd better "get in shape"—whatever that means—so one day I walked over to the park across from our apartment and went for a run. Only a few blocks, just to see how it felt.

I'll tell you how it felt. It was a near-death experience. My lungs nearly exploded. My heart was in my throat, the size of a honeydew. My legs—in complete shock—grew roots. I stumbled home and collapsed on my bed. I was out of breath, out of condition, and out of excuses: How could so little physical exercise make me feel like such a big lump of nothing good?

I somehow survived, loved that first bike trip to France, and came home with a bottomless curiosity to know more about my body and how to keep all its moving parts juiced and happy.

I've always been fascinated by the miracle that is the human body, how it works and plays. I grew up saying I wanted to be a doctor but never took a single pre-med course. After getting a Masters degree in journalism, my first job was in New York as a science writer for Medical World News. But at the time of my Doomsday running experience, I had a dream job at the Chicago Tribune, reviewing movies, theater, TV, and interviewing way too many Hollywood celebrities.

I was also writing feature stories on pretty much whatever interested me, which allowed me many trips to La-La Land in the '70s to research these new things called "holistic health" and "integrative medicine" and the "mind-body connection."

It was all happening in California. In Chicago, in 1976, yoga and yogurt were interchangeable terms and most people considered the mind-body connection another name for the neck.

After a few years of deeper exploration, including a five-part series on Pyramid Power, I went to Mike Argirion, the features editor at the Tribune, and pitched him on a new kind of medical column.

The traditional doctor columns were all about pills and pimples, headaches and hemorrhoids, but I wanted to talk to readers about fitness, wellness, injury prevention, stress reduction, smart eating, deep breathing, and a bunch of other subjects that now fit under the expanding and sustainable umbrella of "healthy lifestyle."

Back then, healthy lifestyle wasn't even a concept. Fitness was just beginning to creep into the consciousness of the nation, right up there with CB radio and needlepoint. Jane Fonda was in leg warmers, going for the burn, Jim Fixx was inspiring a running revolution, farmers markets were just for selling pigs and only tough guys belonged to gyms.

Argirion liked my idea. "Bring me some samples," he said, and immediately I reached out to Dr. David Bachman, team physician for the Chicago Bulls, a highly respected sports medicine doc. Smart, easy-going, open-minded.

"It's a column for people like me," I explained to him, "ordinary mortals who want to live healthier, happier lives and need some sound advice about being active and getting fit without damaging vital parts or giving up red wine."

David liked the idea, too, so we teamed up. I created and wrote the column, and David made sure we were giving out safe, sensible, up-to-date information. It started off in the Tribune's Outside section in September 1976 as a weekly Q&A column and I named it "Dr. Jock" (after Dr. Spock): "I'm a runner with knee pain. What do I do?" Or "How can I lose 10 pounds by Christmas?"

It was a hit in Chicago and soon after became a nationally syndicated column running in dozens of newspapers around the country. David and I did a book together, "Dear Dr. Jock: The People's Guide to Sports and Fitness" (published by E.P. Dutton), and after he moved his practice to the ski mountains of Colorado, I collaborated on the column with Dr. Mitchell Sheinkop, a competitive triathlete and another outstanding sports medicine expert.in Chicago.

Meanwhile, I was becoming a sports medicine expert myself, journalistically speaking, going way beyond the 10,000 hours mark, researching for columns, interviewing doctors and scientists, reading books, taking courses, living the life, and giving lots of healthy lifestyle talks and workshops. In 1996, I became an ACE certified personal trainer, and then a certified Wellcoach many years later. And after 40 years writing what's become America's longest-running fitness column, I've never stopped being curious about what it means to live a vibrant, exciting, healthy, and happy life. (My latest discovery is the standup desk.)

A lot of what I've learned is in this book, 40 chapters with titles that sound like directives but are really just guidelines. If there's one thing I've learned for sure, it's you can't tell another person what to do.

Well, you can, but it doesn't work. It's not an effective way to help people change. And helping women and men and kids of all ages make positive, powerful changes in their lives is at the heart of "All Is Well: The Art {and Science} of Personal Well-Being."

Link Mind and Body. Live a Big, Juicy Life. Be Your Own Uncle Sam. Explore Endlessly. Think In Pictures. Mind Your Menus. Practice De-Aging. Live Long, Die Happy. Some essays will resonate. Others may sound like California dreaming. All are intended to help you discover what *you* personally value when it comes to living your best life, because that's the only way lifelong change is going to happen.

It's up to you, dear reader. I can inform, inspire, educate, amuse, cajole, and otherwise cheer you on, but when push comes to shove—two excellent ways to burn 100 calories—you're in charge of your own personal well-being. And that's the good news because the more you take charge, study up, and stay vigilant, the greater success you'll experience.

As for my successes over the years, and my failures, I am nothing but grateful. I eventually left that dream job at the Tribune to create and produce a nationally syndicated TV series on sports, fitness and adventure called "Energy Express." It ran in 120 cities, won two Emmys, was honored for excellence by the Women's Sports Foundation and NATPE (National Association of Television Programming Executives) and in the early 2000's, I decided to make Energy Express the name of the column too.

I've done many other things in my work life, including running a successful TV production company and having two plays produced, with a third one in the wings. I've performed on camera as the co-host of two TV series, including "Stay Tuned," a never took off rip-off of "Siskel & Ebert & the Movies" but with two TV critics. I am the founding chair of a life-changing nonprofit called Girls in the Game, and I still work as a relentless board member, helping girls get the healthy lifestyle training they need to become strong, powerful women. I was also the managing partner of a startup that staged the world's first Internet auction of independent films, and I wrote and exec produced a documentary in1986 called "Adventure Travel in Israel."

I'll stop now.

The one true red thread that runs through everything I've done and believe in lives on in my ongoing column, and now, this book: Be active. Practice kindness. Eat real food. Live your best life. Be happy. Be grateful. Help others.

All is well.

—Marilynn Preston

Winter

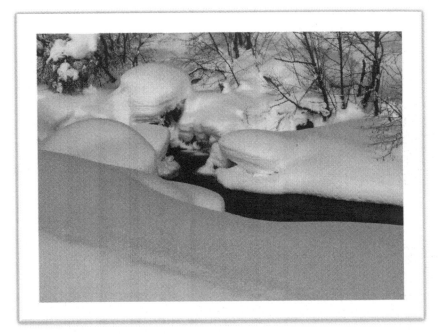

San Juan National Forest, Colorado

"I prefer winter and fall,
when you feel the bone structure of the landscape.
Something wails beneath it,
the whole story doesn't show."
—Andrew Wyeth

"Ten thousand flowers in spring, the moon in autumn,
a cool breeze in summer, snow in winter.
If your mind isn't clouded by unnecessary things,
This is the best season of your life."
—Wu-Men

"Winter spring summer or fall
All you have to do is call
And I'll be there
You've got a friend."
—Carole King

You always remember the First Time. And my first time experiencing the sensational connection between mind and body happened the weekend I turned 30. It was an aikido workshop led by the late, great co-founder of the Human Potential Movement, George Leonard. "Make your arm strong!" he said. I stretched my right arm out, and powered it up, squeezing as hard as I could until it was straight and strong. George pushed slightly, and down it came, like a child, poking at a balloon. Whoa! What just happened? George suggested a visualization. "Now release any tension and imagine you're sending a beam of light through your arm, past your fingers, beyond the wall, down the street..." Strength through relaxation. I was a woman of steel. It was a mind-blowing, life-changing experience. If I can do this, I remember thinking, what else is possible?

Link Mind and Body.

I want to tell you three real-life stories to make one big point about the mind-body connection. It's real. It's not waiting to be proven some day—it *has* been proven, with scientific rigor, time and time again. Your mind and body are communicating with each other right now, inside you, hormonally, chemically, energetically, whether you're aware of it or not.

Becoming aware is a process of self-discovery. All sexes and ages are welcome. When you sense the connections between your thoughts and emotions, and how your body might be expressing them—back pain, indigestion, fatigue—it's a stunning aha! moment.

You won't blame yourself for every illness or accident, but you'll become open to discovering if there are lessons to be learned, especially about the effects of stress on your health, healing and well-being.

True story one: Sandy's husband died some months ago. They'd been together for nearly 25 years, a warm and compatible second marriage for both. Sandy depended on Bill, and Bill depended on Sandy, in a way that made them excited to be with each other, each trying to make the other happier.

Shortly after Bill died, Sandy stumbled and broke her foot. It was agony added to misery and Sandy didn't understand why it happened.

"I know that Bill is watching over me...so why did I have to fall?"

In time, she answered her own question.

"I was moving too fast. I couldn't bear to be in the house without him, so I sold it right away and moved to a smaller place, and I've been making a lot of fast, reckless decisions ever since."

Sandy decided her broken foot was a sign to slow down, move more cautiously. It's not taking away her deep grief, Sandy says, but her mood is better, and she's making smarter decisions.

Story two: Lew is 87, his wife, Bonnie, is 86, and they've been living happily, independently, outside Chicago, in a house they never want to leave. On a recent Sunday night, Bonnie was taken to the hospital because she had difficulty breathing. It's not a new problem but it's a scary one. Lew spent the day with her in intensive care and came home to an empty house. He had some supper, put himself to bed, and woke up after a few hours, unable to move his legs. This had never happened before. Lew called a neighbor, who called 911, and after two days of hospital tests, his doctors could find nothing physical to explain his sudden paralysis.

"I didn't want to go on without her," Lew figured out the next day, after his legs returned to normal. "That's why my legs wouldn't work."

Lew is home now, and so is Bonnie, both grateful to be together again.

"The body is an amazing thing," Lew says. "It knows more than I do."

Story three: A married couple—tired of cold winters and in love with Northern California—went to look for a home in Marin County. They were all super expensive, so the couple decided they'd sell another piece of real estate they owned before buying something new in California.

But then the tireless realtor took them to see the house of their dreams.

"This is it!" they cheered, lost in real estate rapture. "We'll never find a better place!"

They bid on the house without waiting for the other property to sell, which involved a risky bridge loan among other negatives. But what the heck, they high-fived: no guts, no glory.

The night before signing the offer, the wife suddenly felt the worst pain of her life gripping across her chest, lurching down her right arm. She hadn't fallen, lifted weights or done a crooked handstand in yoga.

"Is this a heart attack?" she wondered. " No! It feels deeply muscular, like someone is twisting my arm. "

Her partner jumped to the exact right conclusion.

"We're not buying the house! Look what your body is telling us. If you can't move your right arm, you can't sign the offer. Forget it. We'll wait until the time is right."

The next day the wife saw a wise body worker, fluent in neuromuscular stress, and by noon, her arm was 95 percent better.

And she used it to hug her most understanding partner.

ENERGY EXPRESS-O!　All Is One

"Body is not stiff, mind is stiff."
—K. Pattabhi Jois

GOING DEEPER

Decide for yourself that you want to experience that mind-body connection. There are many paths, but reading about it won't take you there. You need curiosity, an open mind, a teacher and a training that helps you plug into the electrifying flow of energy that develops when your body and mind work in harmony.

Yoga is famous for it. So is training in martial arts, including Qigong, tai chi, aikido, taekwondo, karate. The Alexander Technique can take you there, and so can Feldenkrais, somatics training, and Pilates.

What about fishing? Yes! Hiking in a forest? Absolutely! Posting your 20th tweet of the day? Not so much.

Once you have that felt sense of a body-mind connection, you'll want to keep coming back to it, time and again. It never gets tiresome or boring. Instead, it becomes a way of seeing the interconnectedness of *all* things, inner and outer, humans and rocks, the sea and the stars.

Start where you are. Even if you've never felt the connection before, it is there, waiting for you.

I'm fascinated by change. I've trained to be a Wellcoach to get to the heart of the mystery: How is it that some people can slim down, or sober up, or let go of crippling emotions like anger and guilt, while others stay stuck in the paralyzing groove of woulda, shoulda, coulda? It's more about a readiness to change and less about a will of iron. Positive thinking is a lifesaver. You need to believe you can always begin again.

Begin. Again.

The new year is here. Change is in the air. The making of resolutions is heard in the land, and nearly all of them have to do with living a happier, healthier, more satisfying life:

"I want to start exercising every day!"

"I'm going to lose 20 pounds by Valentine's Day!"

"I want to play more, work less…learn to cook…cut out the sugar and diet sodas…start eating breakfast…restore my '67 Mustang…go to yoga class twice a week, etc."

It's your call, your choice, your personal vision of what your best self looks like a year from now. The work is to create the vision—for yourself, your family, your company—and strive toward it, step by step, some times taking a step back, but always moving forward.

And here's the essential question: If you dream it, can you do it? The answer that serves you best is yes. Like plants turning to the light, we humans are capable of turning our lives around and making smarter choices.

As your most personal trainer, I must tell you that the odds are against you. Statistically, backsliding is to behavior change as slicing is to golf. The mind attaches to the negative. It doesn't like change, actually resists it, and it will invent clever ways to throw you off course. Experts tell us that most people will fail to keep their New Year's resolutions within the first three months.

But here's the good news: You are not most people. You are uniquely you, hard-wired and biochemically organized to change your life in profound ways if and when you are ready.

Genuine and long-lasting lifestyle change is possible. Take it from someone who had a near-death experience at 30 when I tried to run a mile. You must trust in yourself— really! truly! deeply!—because the more you believe you *can* do something, the more likely you *will* do it.

That relationship between belief and action is called self-efficacy, a key concept that enables you to defy the odds and make New Year's resolutions that last, if not a lifetime, at least several nourishing years. And then, as always, you can begin again.

To make change happen in your life, it helps to understand how change happens. For that, please turn to more than 25 years of research by Dr. James Prochaska and colleagues, authors of the classic book "Changing for Good," an excellent guide to help you move from not thinking about change to thinking about it, to planning for it, to doing it, to maintaining the change for a lifetime.

One of Prochaska's pearls (or maybe it's a thorn) is, if you're not ready for change, it won't happen. Don't beat yourself up or waste your time. But when you are ready, it can happen. Obstacles are overcome and single-minded determination kicks in. How do you know if you're ready? Keep reading.

Go inside. You can't quit sugar, lose weight and commit yourself to daily workouts just because your spouse, doctor or insurance company wants you to. You need to dig deep and decide for yourself: Am I truly ready to change? Am I done with the excuses, the drama, the need to feel shame and blame? What are the pros? What are the cons? Write it down. Think it through. If you need coaching help, get it.

When your pros outweigh your cons, you're ready for the next step: Identifying the challenges involved and coming up with specific strategies to overcome them. You can't rush through—or fake—this self-discovery phase. Well, you can... but your lifestyle change will last as long as a bad pedicure.

Set realistic goals. Unrealistic goals—"I'll lose 20 pounds by Valentine's Day!"—set you up for failure. Can you starve, deny, torture yourself? Sure. But it's dumb and teaches you nothing about healthy eating. Scale down your goals to bite-sized, doable challenges—a kitchen makeover, a meatless Monday, two 30-minute walks a week instead of four. The point is to feel successful on a weekly basis. Small victories boost your confidence and motivate you to stay on track.

Be specific or nothing will change. Don't vaguely tell yourself to cut out sweets, for instance. Decide on the details: Snack on seven almonds instead of Almond Joys or switch your morning muffin for a bowl of unsweetened yogurt, walnuts and some blueberries.

If it's physical fun, aka exercise, you want more of, be specific about what you'll do and when. Schedule workouts on your calendar. "Speed walk for 30 minutes around the neighborhood on Tuesday morning, starting at 7 a.m." Details make all the difference!

Slow down; Be patient. Change is not linear. It's often two steps forward, one stumble back. Some days, the best part of your workout is simply showing up. Accept that. New habits take the time they take.

When you feel yourself slipping and falling—and you will!—get back up and begin again. Plan for success. And if you're fooling yourself and unwilling to do the work of change, accept it. For now.

As my favorite Jedi master and wellness coach, Yoda, revealed years ago:

"Do. Or do not. There is no try."

When you're ready to change, you don't try. You do.

ENERGY EXPRESS-O!   Ready, Set, Go.

"People don't resist change. They resist being changed."
—Peter Senge

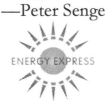

GOING DEEPER

Create a wellness vision for yourself.

Imagine yourself a year from now, living a life that is happier, healthier and more fulfilling, whatever that means to you.

Paint the picture in glorious detail. What, specifically, are you doing? How are you feeling? Are you alone or with other people? Name their names. See their faces. Feel your joy.

Take your time, and when you're finished detailing your wellness vision, write it down and read it back to yourself, out loud. People believe what they hear themselves say, any good wellness coach will tell you. So say it loud, say it proud, and don't get tangled up in judgment. It's your vision, your life, and it will be up to you to make it happen.

Here's an example to inspire you, taken from the wellness vision of a frustrated but determined woman I know who went on to make remarkable changes in her own life.

"I see myself playing with my grandchildren at the beach, and my back pain is gone, and I'm not ashamed of how I look in a swimsuit because I'm having a fabulous time and I feel loved and liberated."

Once you're satisfied with your wellness vision, you'll want a detailed plan to make it happen. If you can team up with a gifted coach, you'll benefit from invaluable support. You'll have to lead the way, but you'll have a partner to dance with, an ally who helps you resolve your ambivalence and build on your strengths.

We don't change because some healthy lifestyle expert comes along and tells us we should. We change when we are ready. Having a wellness vision can help us get ready.

And besides all that, it's just a fun thing to do.

Why is it so hard to slow down and savor the moment? Because the mind is like a monkey, the Buddhists tell us, always jumping from one thing to the next, from the past to the future and back again, bouncing, leaping, the opposite of steady and calm. It's exhausting, and depleting, and the seduction and lure of the 24/7 Internet of Constant Connection isn't helping. But this is our modern world. We are online, on call, on edge and under surveillance many hours a day. What can we do?

Slo-o-o-ow Down.

Are you in a big hurry to slow down?

I am. And I'm not alone. I was just plowing through the 2016 Yoga in America Study—80 pages! Hurry and get to the point!—describing how the popularity of yoga has gone from a wave to a tsunami.

In the U.S., the number of practitioners has lifted into an unassisted handstand, soaring from 20.4 million in 2012 to more than 36 million today.

Some time ago, about 58 of us put our mats down in a huge tent at Esalen, the renowned retreat center devoted to exploring human potential, perched on the spectacular coastline at Big Sur, California. We were there to dive deeply into the Zen of Slowing Down, a five-day workshop led by Tias Little and Henry Shukman.

Keeping it understated, Tias is a master yoga teacher and Henry is a master Zen teacher. They are good friends and students of one another, as well as friends of mine. Their sublime yoga and Zen centers in Santa Fe, New Mexico, are only a mile and a half apart. What a coincidence.

"In an age of acceleration, nothing can be more exhilarating than going slow," Henry reads to us at the start of the week, quoting Pico Iyer.

"In an age of constant distraction, nothing is so luxurious as paying attention.

"In an age of constant movement, nothing is so urgent as sitting still."

Sitting still. Paying attention. Going slow. All that, plus wild waves, passing dolphins and exquisite vegetables pulled out of Esalen's organic garden just that morning and served up at community dinners that have the look, feel and feathers of a Federico Fellini film.

I want to share a few highlights of the workshop, because Tias and Henry have many wise teachings to offer, but first let me assure you that you don't have to go to Esalen or a hermit's cave to begin to slow down your own busy life.

As Henry says—a core truth at the heart of many teachings—"start where you are." Accepting yourself and your life just as they are allows for change to happen, and, from that place, you can begin to let go of haste and an accelerated pace of life that makes your muscles tight, your body sore, your heart constricted.

Paying attention—being in the moment—is a crucial part of slowing down. It can happen anywhere, anytime. When we did walking meditation outside with Henry, it happened by paying strict attention to the soles of our feet.

When you do yoga with Tias Little, the focus is not only on the alignment of the pose but also—always!—on how it feels. The deep somatic work he guides us through at the start of class—on our backs, on our blankets—requires us to direct our awareness to what's going on inside: Is my sacrum level? Can I draw energy up the inside of my legs? Is my heart open wide, my kidneys floating?

If you stop to let your rational mind question, then you've lost the moment of influencing the subtle body, also the title of his latest book. Tias' style of mind-body training—very precise, very playful—enables his students to develop our somatic intelligence. And that—along with a lot of time spreading my sitting bones—has guided me to an understanding of what a profound, self-healing practice yoga can be.

"The everyday world we live in values accomplishment, achieving, acquiring," Henry says, as we all nod and know the truth of that and the stress of that.

We are all scrambling to have the best house, the best job, the best car. "What if we let ourselves be as we are?" Henry asks. "Why hurry up? Why not enjoy the ride?"

Notice pulsating rhythms. Your body is alive with pulsating rhythms as energy flows in your cells, brain, joints, muscles and tissues. Tias tells us that if we can slow down enough to tune in—through yoga, breathing and meditation—we can help the body heal, stay healthy and even glow.

"It's like a light shining from within," he quotes Ged Sumner and Steve Haines. "It's the glow of life that can be seen in the skin, eyes and the aura."

Fear not, dear reader! You don't have to believe in your aura to go for the glow. It's what vibrant health looks like. You might see it in the mirror one day, and slowing down is one deeply satisfying way to make it happen.

For more on the transformative ways of Tias and Henry, check out their websites, prajnayoga.com and mountaincloud.org.

As for Esalen, it's the best place on earth to learn to float your kidneys.

ENERGY EXPRESS-O!   Other Worldly

"I have lived with several Zen masters—all of them cats."
—Eckhart Tolle

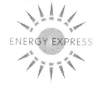

GOING DEEPER

Do a walking meditation. No experience necessary.
Here's a summary of Henry's step-by-step teaching:
Step 1. Walk into nature. Sometimes walking meditation is done inside a Zen temple—a break from long periods of sitting meditation—but doing it outside, in nature, offers special benefits. Wear comfortable shoes and appropriate clothes, and pick a path that is safe and unencumbered.

Step 2: Arrange your hands. There is a Zen way of doing just about everything—from eating a meal to being with your dog—so it's no surprise that walking meditation in Henry's Sanbo-Zen lineage has rules about how to hold your hands.

"You put your right hand around your right thumb and use the left hand to gently press your right hand against your solar plexus, just below the diaphragm, the energetic center of strength, confidence and joy," Henry demonstrated. "That's the Zen way."

Is it the only way? Of course not. It's so not-Zen to dictate to people what they can and can't do.

Step 3: Mind your posture. Walking meditation needn't be reminiscent of a funeral march. Follow the rules, but you can also follow your bliss. Walk mindfully, in silence, with an upright spine and a slight chin tuck. Your eyes are open and lowered, but not in a way that makes your walking unsafe. Personally, I like to throw in a serene smile. Walk in a way that feels relaxed and aware, opening up the deepest channels of the body, allowing for a flow of energy up and down the spine, drawing up from the earth, drawing down from the sky. I know it sounds a little woo-woo, but so what? Lots of things that used to seem woo-woo are now known to be true-true.

Step 4: Don't focus on your breath. Really? "Let your mind rest in the soles of your feet," Henry told us. Don't overthink it. Just let go and let it happen, walking at a comfortable pace, focusing your mind's eye on the bottom of your feet.

When you lose focus—and you will, just like in sitting meditation—you simply acknowledge the lapse, congratulate yourself for noticing, return your awareness to the soles of your feet, and keep it there until your walk is finished.

Step 5: Nothing to gain. At the end of our refreshing and revelatory 20-minute walking meditation, Henry explained a little more about its power.

"It's about being as we are, where we are...the experience of the now. Our minds grasp for meaning, grasp for understanding…

"There is nothing to understand," said Henry, "There is just now."

Many people hibernate in winter. I can't bear the thought. I grew up on the South Side of Chicago (rhymes with Dr. Zhivago) and I used to hate the cold. Brrr-rrr-rr-r! Hunched shoulders, frozen smile, bad attitude. But once I began to relax and embrace winter, rather than fighting and resisting, I started looking forward to snowflakes and icicles. Learning to layer helped a lot. So did learning to ski. And when I discovered snowshoeing, I was in bliss. So, this winter, put on a wild Turtle Fur hat and find the winter sport that calls to you, or at least, doesn't kill you.

Go Play in the Snow.

My friend's son just broke several moving parts in a snowboarding accident. It was serious. He'll spend months in rehab and his stressed-out parents will spend thousands in medical fees.

Jake's a smart kid, a sophomore in college, athletic and strong. It turns out he was a big fan of the Winter Olympics and spent hours watching all those champion snowboarders do their somersaults, twists and 360 big spins.

Awesome! Cool! Grab it, Shaun!

When Jake had his chance to go snowboarding, he pretty much lost his mind. Maybe his helmet was too tight. He decided to try a simple kick flip. No big deal, he thought. It's a beginner trick. He'd seen it done hundreds of times.

Of course, it was an insane move on his part. No training. No coaching. Just Jake and his brand-new Burton sliding down a mountain in Colorado, young and fearless and hoping for the best.

The best thing that happened is that he lived.

The flip side of Jake's story involves Janet, a woman I met recently at a fundraiser for old growth forests. She, too, was inspired by the Winter Olympics. After a few nights of watching the skaters, she decided to go back to figure skating. After a 50-year hiatus. She loved skating when she was a kid, but gave it up to live her grown-up life, enjoy her family and, over time, gain about 35 pounds.

"I was watching Kim Yuna...and all of a sudden, something inside of me called out." she told me. "I can do that! I used to do that! I want to do it again!" She felt a shift, and she acted on it.

Janet's joined a skating club and has taken eight lessons. She's sleeping better, feeling perkier and—oh, yes—she's gone from a size 14 to a 12 without even trying.

Have you found your cold-weather sport yet? If yes, what are you doing this winter to get better at it? Learning new things builds your brain, and your confidence.

If you don't have a winter sport, what are you waiting for? (Nope, the answer isn't "summer.") Get outside, get moving, see what all the excitement's about. Hibernation—so good for bears, so not good for humans—tends to layer on the pounds and depress the spirit.

How to find your winter sport. This is our interactive moment. Let your mind play with the question: What winter sport calls to you? Snowshoeing? Cross-country skiing? Don't be ashamed to say curling.

Once you have your answer, make your move. Take a lesson. Join a club. Listen to that inner voice. It's the healthiest part of you, longing to breathe hard and feel the exhilaration and joy of being outdoors in the snow and ice, having your best time. And it's so *beautiful* out there.

Learn to layer. Dressing for cold weather workouts is simple once you understand the basics of layering. The garment closest to your skin should be a nontoxic material that wicks away your moisture, your sweat. That means give up your cottons. When cotton gets wet, it stays wet and that can make you feel cold and uncomfortable when the temperature drops. The top layer depends on how active you will be. Some downhill skiers wear down. A cross-country skier would faint in a heavy down jacket. Just make sure your top-layer jacket is waterproof and wind-resistant.

Cross-country vs. downhill. Skiing is a magnificent sport in all its forms, but there are big differences between cross-country and downhill. Cross-country is aerobic and will boost your fitness. Do it long enough and often enough, and it will get you into the shape of your life. That's not true of downhill skiing, which is really a controlled fall. To ski well and safely, you need to develop strength and flexibility off the slopes.

Downhill also costs a lot more than cross-country. Both sports offer plenty of thrills, chills, magic. Whichever you choose, prepare with sport-specific training to develop balance and flexibility, take lessons and bring your mind into play.

If you're still turning a cold shoulder to being outdoors in winter—throwing another log on the fire as you read this—accept that, and keep moving indoors. Save your money and buy one piece of home fitness gear—a stationary bike, a rower, an elliptical cross trainer—that'll keep you in a sweat till you see your first robin.

ENERGY EXPRESS-O! Laugh at the Cold

"The problem with winter sports is that—follow me closely here—they generally take place in winter."
—Dave Barry

GOING DEEPER

Plan a day of winter-sport wackiness with family and friends. Try to find a physical activity no one's done before.

What would be pure fun? Tubing? Ice fishing? Snow-person building?

I'll never forget playing my one and only round of Goofy Golf in the North Woods. I was dressed in multicolored down from head to toe, it was way below zero, and there was three feet of snow on the ground. We stood on an old used tire, teed up a bright yellow golf ball, and swung away into the frozen wilderness with vintage clubs that hadn't seen the inside of a golf bag in decades. What a hoot!

And yes, it involved a bar.

If you want your life to change, it's good to think out of the box. And for that, we read great thinkers. They can shift our perspective and inspire our own creative thinking. Henry David Thoreau is certainly a role model for sparking our inner explorer. So are Seneca and Anne Lamott. Here are all three, with some superb advice about living your best, most authentic life.

Live a Big, Juicy Life.

My research shows that tens of millions of people make New Year's resolutions concerning their health. By the end of January, you can fit in a Fiat 500 all the people still on track, getting to the gym, walking the stairs, giving up diet colas.

Relax. Finger pointing and guilt mongering, while still part of my cultural heritage, are wildly counterproductive when it comes to lasting lifestyle change. In fact, I have good news for you: Failing to stick to a resolution may not be your fault. It could be the resolution.

Maybe it's too shallow for you. You might do better latching on to a genius's resolution, one that takes you deeper, and leads you to real growth and lasting transformation.

"At the start of each year, humanity sets to better itself as we resolve to eradicate our unhealthy habits and cultivate healthy ones," writes Maria Popova, on her splendid website, Brain Pickings.

Popova explains that while resolutions about better health are the most typical, "the most meaningful ones aim at a deeper kind of health through the refinement of our

mental, spiritual and emotional habits—which often dictate
our physical ones."

Here are three of my favorites from her list. If you see
one you like more than "Zumba class twice a week," go for
it. You've got a whole new year to make it stick:

**"Walk and Be More Present."—Henry David
Thoreau**

It's one thing to tell yourself you'll walk more. It's a
leap forward to challenge yourself to stay in the moment as
you walk, without phoning or listening to music, without
your mind straying to some issue in the past or future. How
do you do it? Focus on your breath. Pay attention to sound.
Feel the soles of your feet as you take every step. Why
bother? Because, as Thoreau explained 150 years ago, in an
essay on the spiritual value of walking, walking without
presence of mind is a missed opportunity to feed the soul
and connect to your essential wildness. No wonder we still
read and quote him.

"I am alarmed when it happens that I have walked a
mile into the woods bodily, without getting there in spirit,"
he wrote.

Where's your spirit when you walk? To affect your
deeper health, resolve to Be Here Now. I find this works
even outside the woods.

**"Make Your Life Wide Rather Than Long."—
Seneca**

"It is not that we have a short time to live," Seneca
wrote about 2,000 years ago, "but that we waste a lot of it."
And he didn't even have TV!

Many of us coast through our lives, "in a trance of
passivity and busyness—the greatest distractions from
living," Popova writes, "mistaking the doing for the being."

Seneca agrees. In his treatise, "On The Shortness Of Life," he writes, "Putting things off is the biggest waste of life."

Don't squander your time, he advises, because you never know how much you have. "The whole future lies in uncertainty; live immediately."

What if you resolved to "live immediately"? What are you putting off for later that would make your life richer and more satisfying right now?

"Let Go of Perfectionism."—Anne Lamott

"Perfectionism is the voice of the oppressor, the enemy of the people," Lamott writes in her classic "Bird by Bird" book about writing, and life.

That inner voice, telling you *you're* not good enough, "will keep you very scared and restless your whole life if you do not awaken and fight back. "

And how do you fight back? Make a lot of mistakes, she writes. Fall on your butt more often. And this: "Put something on your calendar that you know you'll be terrible at," Lamott advises, "like dance lessons, or a meditation retreat. "Don't be so strung out on perfectionism and people pleasing that you forget to have a big juicy, creative life."

What if you resolved to have a bigger, juicier, more creative life this year? What would that look like?

And please don't go looking for outside help on this; it's purely personal. Want to play drums? Read in ancient Greek? Learn to jump rope? Forget being perfect. Be forgiving to yourself instead, and see where enthusiasm, curiosity and grace take you.

ENERGY EXPRESS-O!   Let the Light In

"Ring the bells that still can ring
"Forget your perfect offering
"There is a crack in everything
"That's how the light gets in."
—Leonard Cohen

GOING DEEPER

Sign up for something—this week!—that you've always wanted to do but haven't so far because you always find a reason that gets in the way. No time, no money, no one to go with, no way to get there...

Just say no to all that, remembering that the mind attaches to the negative. That's the default. Pay no attention and refocus on finding a way to live your dream, even a little one.

What'll it be? Drumming? Square dancing? Raising poodles?

Take a positive step forward—this moment!—to aim high and go deep. Why wait?

It's one thing to lose my mitten or my umbrella, but losing my mind sounds unbearable. That's one reason I'm such a student of neuroscience and the remarkable discoveries of the last 40 years. One difficult truth we're facing is the impact of unlimited distraction on the human brain. Is technology moving us forward in our thinking or is it pulling us away from the kind of quiet reflective time the brain needs to make sense of our world and our best place in it? The pace of life is so much quicker, while destructive plaque grows so much thicker, so it's up to us to keep our precious brains juiced and jubilant for as long as we can.

Grow Your Gray Matter.

Every 67 seconds, someone in America develops Alzheimer's disease.

When I read this terrifying fact, it stuck in my brain the way you remember your first root canal or your last car crash.

(Why can't I remember where I read that study? Think! Is this a sign of age-related mental decline? If I sit here long enough, will it come back to me?)

Get me to the running path. Brain breaks are mandatory at Healthy Lifestyle U, where you're taught to include time in your day to walk, run, bike, dance or garden, all admirable ways to stop worrying about your memory and remember this: There are things *you can do* to boost your brain power, to take advantage of its neuroplasticity. If you eat right and treat it right, your brain can grow and develop in wonderful ways, no matter your age. Senility may happen—life is a mystery—but scientifically speaking, it's less likely to happen if you have a plan of action.

Grow your gray matter. The research is in, again and again: Physical activity is essential when it comes to growing your gray matter, particularly in those regions of the brain responsible for memory and higher-level thinking.

(An example of higher-level thinking would be tossing out all products with artificial sweeteners.)

According to a significant new study published in the Journal of Alzheimer's Disease, brain scan studies now confirm what neuroscientists have been telling us for ages: Physical activity can prevent and postpone mental decline in aging brains. It can even substantially reduce the risk of Alzheimer's. Imagine that. No magic pills, no fetal-lamb-cell smoothies. Just you and your body in motion, a few times a week. The researchers aren't talking about hardcore, super-strenuous workouts. Nope. Even recreational amounts of cycling, walking and pulling weeds make a big difference when it comes to keeping your marbles.

Eat smart. I'm not a fan of diet as a verb, but there are certain types of diets-as-a-noun that are worth discussing.

The latest for brain health is the MIND diet, developed by researchers at Rush University Medical Center in Chicago.

The MIND diet is the love child of the DASH diet (targeted for lowering blood pressure) and the gold-standard Mediterranean diet. Besides blueberries, for the antioxidants, it also wants you to eat healthy fats such as salmon, nuts and olive oil.

Why? Because they are the fats your body needs to stay in balance and combat inflammation. Nonfat products, which are mostly fake foods, don't do that. I know it's counterintuitive—as in, "Doesn't fat make you fat?"—but the bottom line is, nutrition-wise, you can't fool Mother Nature. Well, you can for a while, but she will probably mess with your brain and make you gain weight.

Mind your greens. The MIND diet also includes eating leafy greens. Rush University researchers found that people who ate two servings a day had the cognitive ability of someone 11 years younger. Eleven years younger! Talk about nuts.

It's crazy to think how much money the country could save if citizens started making healthy food choices instead the ones pushed in brilliant, funny and ultimately sickening commercials.

"Alzheimer's is the most expensive disease in the country," says the Alzheimer's Association, advertising these days on Politico, where I hope they are getting through to decision-makers.

"Every hour, Alzheimer's costs the country $18.3 million dollars. Today, Alzheimer's costs the country $236 billion a year and that will quadruple to more than $1 trillion over the next generation."

That blows my mind. A trillion dollars ain't chicken feed, which is also likely to be a cause of Alzheimer's, but I digress.

Control your devices. I know small-screen monitoring and engagement is pretty irresistible, but discretion is required if you want a strategy to save your brain. We've been ignoring the warnings for years. A 2005 study in the journal Brain and Cognition found that for people between the ages of 40 and 59, the risk of Alzheimer's went up 1.3 times with every added hour of TV they watched per day. Twelve years later, even babies are growing up with tiny TVs in their cribs. A terrible idea!

Whereas the real Baby Einstein, Alfred that is, grew up playing outside.

We are dependent on our devices for more and more, diving deeper and more continuously into the invisible soup of small-screen brain disturbance. And I'm not even mentioning the physical effects on our brains of all that incoming radiation. If you think Big Sugar has been keeping the truth from us about the health damage that comes from too much sugar, wait until the Big Phone industry gets the scrutiny it deserves. But I digress.

Want to combat your own technology overload? First, pry yourself away from all your distractive devices. Then wander over to a quiet spot—indoors or out, in a chair or on a cushion—and meditate for some time.

ENERGY EXPRESS-O!   Uncommon Sense

"Everybody gets so much information all day long that they lose their common sense."
—Gertrude Stein

GOING DEEPER

Practice prevention. There are all sorts of brain activities you can do to stay sharper, longer, and live a more engaged, invigorated life.

Doing crossword puzzles makes you better at doing crossword puzzles, and playing bridge makes you a better bridge player, and both can contribute to a healthier, happier brain.

What else? Learn a language. Memorize a new poem every week. Take up a new sport. Travel to places you've never been. Take a different route home or to work.

Your brain likes it when new neural pathways are created, when synapses connect that never wired or fired together before.

Dancing–on your own, with a partner—can do that. So can curling up with a good book, or growing your own food, or pulling a mix of things out of your fridge and making something curiously edible for dinner.

Your brain thrives on challenge, on spontaneity, on the unpredictable. And if none of those are readily available, find the dark chocolate.

I've always been a shameless cheerleader for adventure travel. And I still walk the talk every chance I get. My biggest, tallest, longest challenge was in 2000, an amazing, life-changing six-week trek through Nepal and Tibet that included a circumambulation of Mount Kailash—not the highest mountain in the world but said to be the holiest. The day the yak just ahead of me slipped off the trail and tumbled into the valley was a startling lesson in overcoming fear. (The yak survived. Me, too.) The continuing boom in adventure travel is one of the most thrilling healthy lifestyle trends of the last 40 years, right up there with the revolution in women's sports and the rise of organic everything.

Explore Endlessly.

Show me a backpack, and my toes start to tingle. I've been dog-sledding in Lapland, rafting in Costa Rica, bicycling in France, scuba diving in Mexico, sailing in Greece—I'll stop now—and the more adventures I take, the more enthusiastic I am about recommending them to others. Others being you, dear reader.

Why? Because active vacations are what joy feels like. They are challenging, totally distracting and sometimes life changing. Best of all, they lure you into nature, where all the good stuff happens.

Mountains, rivers, forests, underwater caves—nature soothes and heals in a way that the blackjack tables at Caesar's Palace never can. When you challenge yourself outdoors—physically, mentally, emotionally—you discover new things about yourself. When I went around Mount Kailash, for instance, I learned I could take a pee in a plastic bag instead of crawling outside the tent into the bone-chilling cold and snow of 17,000 feet.

My favorite kind of adventure is the one I've never had before, which is why I leaped at the chance to go whale watching in winter in warm and sunny Baja Mexico.

It wasn't just whale watching—it was amazingly close encounters with big blue whales, the largest animals to ever live on Earth, even bigger than the dinosaurs.

And it wasn't just the blue whales; it was also a week of inspired yoga with two of my favorite teachers, Tias and Surya Little.

And it wasn't just deep breathing and oceanic meditation; it was time on the water with a wildly enthusiastic whale expert named, of all things, Michael Fishbach, founder of Eco-Interactions.

"These guys are a complete mystery," Michael says about his pals, the big blues, after more than 20 years of research. "Why do they keep coming back to Baja? When do they give birth? And where? There's so much we really don't know."

What we do know about the big blue whales is mind-boggling. They weigh up to 150 tons. The heart of a blue whale is the size of a Volkswagen beetle, and their arteries are large enough for a child to crawl through. They can swim at speeds up to 30 mph, can dive down to 10,000 feet and can hold their breath up to an hour. The average length is 70 to 85 feet, but they can grow to 100 feet or more. Their life span is thought to be 60 to 70 years. They eat up to four tons of krill a day—tiny, shrimp-like creatures—hold the cocktail sauce.

Here's the sad part—they are a seriously endangered species. Thanks to illegal whaling, pollution, fishing nets, cargo ships, and killer whales, there are only about 10,000 blue whales left on the planet, which is why Michael and some colleagues started the Great Whale Conservancy under the umbrella of Earth Island Institute.

You can do your part by visiting the Earth Island Institute website and learning about his campaign, but the best way to get a feeling for what magnificent beasts they are is to do what I was lucky enough to do, and go out with Michael at 6 in the morning on the Sea of Cortez—with the full moon setting on one side of the bay and the fiery Mexican sun rising on the other. And watch for spouts. And just listen.

"HHH-A-A-AUhhhh!" is my lame attempt to repeat a sound I'll never forget—the exhalation of a big blue whale rising to the surface to take a breath. Wow. How can I explain? The blues have a *presence*.

Energetically, you feel a mysterious connection to an extraordinary being. When they fluke—their huge tails rising high in the air as they dive deep—it feels like a blessing. Blues are notoriously calm and trusting, neither threatened nor threatening, and their brains function on a higher level than many of our elected officials.

Some of the 20 to 30 blue whales we saw came within 15 feet of our little boat. So close! I gasped in amazement. I imagined myself on their backs, diving deep into my own fears of the sea. I felt inexplicably overwhelmed with joy and gratitude. This never happened to me at Disney World.

ENERGY EXPRESS-O!   Find Your Inner Traveler

"The biggest adventure you can ever take is to live the life of
your dreams."
—Oprah Winfrey

ENERGY EXPRESS

GOING DEEPER

This week, sit down and dream up your ideal adventure vacation.

Then plan it.

Then do it.

If you feel fearful or anxious, witness it, accept it...and stick to the plan.

The best adventures begin when you let go of what's holding you back.

When you return home, go through your photos and make a book. Include your feelings and fears, your trials and triumphs.

Who did you bond with?

What challenges appeared and how did you meet them?

When were the best parts?

Where are you going next year?

Meditation is trendy. Meditation is cool. Meditation in the workplace. Meditation in school. (I feel like I'm channeling Dr. Seuss.) I believe the mainstreaming of meditation as one of the most uplifting developments of the last 40 years. In this essay on the benefits of sitting still and witnessing whatever comes up, I'm happy to introduce you to the work of a well-known meditation master, Sharon Salzberg. I've described her as a cross between Roseanne Barr and the Dalai Lama, and I mean that in the nicest, kindest way.

Meditate on This.

Before "Real Happiness," Sharon Salzberg's book about creating a more joyful life, she experienced real unhappiness and deep despair.

Her father left home when she was four. Her mother died when she was nine. She went to live with her grandparents, but her grandfather died soon after. Her father returned, tried to kill himself and ended up a mental patient for the rest of his life. And you think you had a tough childhood?

By the time Sharon left for college, she'd lived in five different households, all chaotic and confusing. She felt abandoned and angry. And then, when she was 18— convinced she was unworthy of love—Sharon went to India. And her life changed in wonderful ways.

Sharon learned to meditate, to look deep within. And what she discovered is what she's been living and teaching every since: that goodness exists in everyone, that she is wildly worthy of love, that everyone deserves to be happy, and that everyone can be happy, once you learn to be mindful, compassionate, and free of judgments.

"If you can breathe, you can meditate," she writes in "Real Happiness: The Power of Meditation," a terrific how-to guide that includes audio of Sharon's sultry tones, expertly narrating nine guided meditations.

As co-founder of the Insight Meditation Society, she's been teaching her style of Buddhist-based meditation for more than 35 years, and in this book, her eighth, she's stripped away all the esoteric Buddhist text and terms and gone straight to the heart of the teachings.

"Once we have a sense of a center," she writes, "we can more easily withstand the onslaught of overstimulation, uncertainty and anxiety the world launches at us, without getting overwhelmed."

I heard Sharon explore the power of meditation at a Real Happiness retreat at the Upaya Institute and Zen Center in Santa Fe, New Mexico. It's a think tank for going beyond thinking, and the founder, Joan Halifax Roshi, my friend of many years, has a well-deserved reputation for presenting world-class teachers.

Sharon fits the bill. She's funny, smart, and a gifted storyteller, with a soothing voice and surprisingly sleepy eyes. Her no-big-deal, anyone-can-do-it approach to meditation is gentle, inviting, and entirely profound.

If you want to learn, or you're curious to know what's involved, Sharon has come up with 28-day program, step by step, story by story, breath by breath. Without judgment, and with humor, she points the way toward a life of compassion, connection, and loving kindness, while teaching the skills to let go of fear, anger, and envy.

At the end of day one, I bought three copies of her book for friends.

(I could have bought 30.) Here are a few highlights from her talks:

Meditation isn't a religion. You don't have to be Buddhist or Hindu or a yogi to practice. The techniques Sharon teaches can be done within any faith tradition or be done in an entirely secular way. You don't need special skills or a huge chunk of time every day. (She recommends twenty minutes, but if you've only got five, start there.) Meditation is not an attempt to stop thinking, she says. It's "a way to recognize our thoughts, to observe and understand them, and relate to them more skillfully."

Why practice meditation? Meditation is a medical miracle. Clinical studies show it promotes wellness, reduces stress, boosts learning and memory, improves sleep and depression, lowers blood pressure and much more. Sharon focuses more on the emotional and psychological benefits: learning how to stay in the moment, letting go of judgments, becoming aware of a calm and stable center that gets us through tough times.

Meditation isn't passive, she says. "Deepening our concentration brings us power and energy and healing."

Losing focus is normal. Sharon's taught thousands of people to meditate, and the one truth we all need to hear, over and over, is that losing concentration is normal. It happens to everyone. You start out focusing on your breath, and after just a few inhales and exhales, you're thinking about lunch, or your itchy nose, or a new app for organizing all your other apps. No problem, says Sharon. Just start over again, without a moment of shame or frustration.

And what if you feel bored, restless, deep sadness when you attempt to meditate?

"A difficult session is just as valuable as a pleasant one—maybe more so," she knows. "We can look mindfully at joy, sorrow or anguish. It doesn't matter what's going on; transformation comes from changing our relationship to what's going on."

It's as simple as that. Hah!

ENERGY EXPRESS-O!   Let Go of the Struggle

"Your goal is not to battle with the mind, but to witness the mind."
—Swami Muktananda

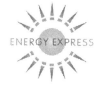

GOING DEEPER

Sit.

If your body can sit comfortably on a cushion in a classic, cross-legged posture, go for it. It's impressive, but not necessary.

Being impressive is also not necessary.

If you prefer to sit quietly on a chair, or a kneeling stool, that's fine, too.

Start where you are.

Focus inside, and examine your ideas about meditation.

Don't judge. Don't make up stuff. Just explore.

Do you think it's all hocus-pocus?

Are you totally gung-ho because it cured your back pain and led you to your soul mate?

Would you like to try meditation but honestly can't sit still long enough to learn?

Meditate on whatever thoughts and feelings arise. If nothing arises, try not to fall asleep.

After a while, come back to your breath, and let it all go.

Don't worry about whether you did this little exercise right.

Just doing it is doing it right.

*As your most personal trainer—ACE certified since 1996—
I confess it's been wildly frustrating to wait around for
mainstream health care in America to dramatically
improve. There is progress, but it's still a broken-down,
who-cares-about-prevention, for-profit business. The
bottom-line financial health of drug companies,
insurance companies, and manufacturers of processed
foods matters more to policymakers than the overall
health and wellness of We the People. When you know
that, you know everything. And you can adjust.*

Take Care of Yourself.

"If I am not for myself, who will be for me?" said
Hillel the Elder, a wise teacher who lived in Jerusalem
around the time B.C. became A.D.

That's the essence of self-care. It's not selfish; it's
sensible. When you decide to be in charge of your own
health and wellness—staying active, eating well, getting
enough sleep, doing practices that calm your mind and revive
your spirit—everyone you know, including your pets, will
benefit.

Hillel, again:

"Take care of yourself," he said. "You never know
when the world will need you."

And now the hop, skip, and a jump to sports injury
prevention. People who lead active lives risk injuries. That's
the truth. We twist our backs or strain our shoulders or a lot
worse, and the cost in terms of health care dollars spent and
work hours lost can be crippling.

As a self-caring person, there is a lot you can do to
avoid sports injuries. That's what I want to focus on, because

prevention is still the runt of the litter when it comes to U.S. health care, and you can't practice what you don't know.

Sure, accidents will happen—you turn your ankle sliding into second base, you pinch your finger on the bicycle bell—but the more you understand the basics of self-care, the prouder Hillel will be of you.

Don't overdo it. Overuse injuries are the most common sports injuries. They pop up in different disguises—back pain, sore shins, strained knees—but the cause is the same: You're doing too much, too soon, with a body that isn't strong or flexible enough to take the stress. You have to back off to move forward. And if you're working with a bully of a trainer who pushes you too hard, screaming "no pain, no gain," get yourself a more evolved coach.

Develop body awareness. To lower your risk of injury—any injury—learn some basic anatomy so that you can sense your body, listen to your body, even talk back to your body, giving new meaning to "I've Got You Under My Skin."

Before you put yourself in motion—at work or play— take a few moments to scan your whole body, from your cranium to your callouses. When you sense tension—a stiff neck, tight shoulders, hips that hurt when you walk—relax and release, a mind-body trick that is easier said than done, but always worth the effort. Then bathe the area with fresh revitalizing breath.

This concept of tuning into your inner self may sound a little woo-woo, but it's a state of body awareness that I urge you to develop. Qigong, yoga, meditation, mindfulness, and somatics training can take you down that path, and so can a terrific book I'm constantly reading called "Awakening Somatic Intelligence" by Risa F. Kaparo, Ph.D. Fascinating!

Slow down. If you're concerned about getting hurt playing sports, know it's OK to slow down. Slow walking. Conscious running. Yin yoga. You don't have to go fast to get into shape, physically or mentally.

In fact, when you slow down your movement, you have time to zone in on what's going on with your muscles, your joints, your breath...and it's this feedback that tells you when to ease off, when to speed up. If you can nip a sports injury in the bud—before it ends up needing a doctor, tests, drugs—you save yourself a whole lot of aggravation, money and time.

Focus and breathe. If your mind wanders and you lose focus when you work out—pondering the past, worrying about the future, texting in between—stupid accidents happen more easily.

Listening to your breath can help keep you focused. Learn to breath fully, deeply, rhythmically. Not only will this focus lower your risk of injury, it's also a good way to release tension and create stability so your body can move more easily, with greater flow.

The opposite of conscious breathing is holding your breath. It can happen easily when you're concentrating on a difficult move, but it's a no no for any sport. And, it's especially risky when it comes to lifting and lowering heavy weights because it can push your blood pressure way too high.

Balance your work out. Muscle imbalance—strong quads but weak hamstrings, a ripped 10-pack in front but tightness and weakness in your lower back—is a common cause of sports injuries. Learn to work your body in a balanced way, front and back, side to side, top to bottom.

Check your gear. Sometimes sports injuries result from a mismatch between you and your equipment: a bike seat that's too low, a tennis racket that's too heavy, 10-year-old running shoes. Your gear should support and fit your body. If you suspect it doesn't, talk to an expert to make sure you're not setting yourself up for injuries down the line.

ENERGY EXPRESS-O! DIY

"If we don't change, we don't grow. If we don't grow, we aren't really living."
—Gail Sheehy

GOING DEEPER

Study anatomy. Your own. It's an unusual but highly effective way to promote your own health and healing.

You don't have to memorize anything. You are your own final exam.

Just explore and embrace a Big Picture understanding of where your vital organs are including your heart, your lungs, your kidneys, your colon. Investigate the exquisite architecture of your body, including major bones, vital tendons and ligaments, more than 600 muscles. Learn how your body is constructed, connected, and how it works.

All the while, learn to listen your body. Talk to it, too. Sensation is the language of the body. If you feel jumpy or joyful, tight or terrific, your body is telling you something you need to hear. Pay attention now, or pay a doctor later.

Knowing your anatomy will help you befriend your body. It's a mystery and a miracle, and the sooner you start a dialogue, the sooner you will be taking charge, making change, and nurturing body and mind with your breath.

I know Hillel would approve.

How you age matters. There are zillions of books out there to help you age gracefully, wildly, mindfully, with or without Botox. But what about de-aging, what Kazuaki Tanahashi calls the "Miracle of Each Moment"? Kaz has inspired me time and time again with his gorgeous calligraphy, his boundless enthusiasm for poetry and peace. He's ageless, I remember thinking soon after we met. And now I know why.

Practice De-Aging.

I have a friend visiting me on this small, remote Greek island where I live several months a year. He is a Zen teacher, translator, artist, author and a world-class peace activist. His name is Kazuaki Tanahashi. Sometimes, when people say to him, "Hello. How are you?" Kaz will laugh and answer, "I am de-aging."

In his 80s now, Kaz is the inventor of de-aging. It's not a product or a program. It's a concept, a way of slowing down the aging process without resorting to desperate anti-aging measures involving pills, plastic surgery or fetal lamb cells.

"Anti-aging is defensive thinking," Kaz explains to me one day after breakfast, sitting in our room with a view, overlooking an endless sea. "De-aging is more active. Each moment we have a choice."

Kaz takes a breath, and so do I. I've heard him talk about de-aging before. This time, I'm taking notes.

"The idea is we lose vitality and gain vitality each moment. Aging is not a one-way street, going downhill. We become older, we become younger, every moment."

Kaz has explained his quantum physics-based de-aging theory to many friends who are doctors, and they all agree it's a good one.

"We age as a whole," Kaz continues, his long scraggly beard waving in the breeze. "Our body, our mind...we can't reverse it. But when we look at aging at the micro level—each day, each hour, each moment—we see that it goes up and down. So in each moment, we have a choice."

The choice is between doing something that ages us, or de-ages us, something that makes us more vital or less vital, more healthy or less healthy. He mentions eating well and exercising. (I feel a wellness column writing itself in my mind, which means I'll be free to spend the afternoon de-aging at my favorite beach. I am choosing to be happy.)

"If I'm tired, I can choose to take a walk, or I can watch TV," he elaborates. "I can choose to relax and meditate, or I can smoke. I can overwork, or I can rest. I can take a job that is more stressful or less stressful...and in this way, we can shape our life. Are we aging or are we de-aging? It's an active choice."

When it comes to living a healthier, happier lifestyle, it always comes down to personal choices.

Fortunately for all of us, you don't have to be a Zen master to figure it out. Will you have a donut and diet cola for breakfast or yogurt and fresh fruit? Hold onto anger or let it go? Choose to drive or walk or bike?

"You can't really control overall aging," Kaz says, "but by doing de-aging, we can slow it down."

So de-aging is a kind of practice, I say. Kaz doesn't pick up on the word practice. I feel myself aging, just a little.

What are some other ways we can de-age? I ask.

"It's important to be excited about life!" Kaz says, raising his voice to just above a whisper. "Being in love! You could be in love with art, grandchildren or doing service work. Have a passion. Love what you do!"

Kaz says he loves what he does—writing, painting, running a revolutionary nonprofit called A World Without Armies—but he is aware of his tendency to do too much, for too long.

"I am Japanese; I'm a kind of workaholic. I have to tell myself to slow down, to be lazy. Lazy people don't have to be reminded to be lazy." He stops to laugh at his own joke. "To be lazy doesn't mean not to work. It means to slow down, do less work and be more effective. That kind of laziness."

Negative emotions get in the way of de-aging, Kaz goes on. "Anger, envy, jealousy, hatred...all these negative emotions contribute to aging. So you have to find a way to turn a negative situation into something positive. This is the practice of being calm, more compassionate, more understanding. This turns aging into de-aging"

It's time to take a break, another form of de-aging practice. Can I call it a practice even if Kaz does not?

It's something to think about as I sit on the sand, building a tower out of stones, slowly balancing one little rock at a time, watching myself grow younger every moment.

ENERGY EXPRESS-O!   Zen and Now

"Be open to all teachers, and all teachings,
and listen with your heart."
—Ram Dass

GOING DEEPER

If de-aging is your goal, what will you choose to do differently?

Some possibilities:

—Slow down.

—Give up road rage.

—Get more sleep.

—Join a local singing group.

—Tutor a child.

—Rescue a poodle and take it for walks twice a day.

—Work less, play more, no guilt allowed.

—Turn off your mobile at mealtime.

—Take every single day and moment of your vacation.

—_____ (fill in the blank)

De-aging is all about the choices you make, every day, day by day, day in, day out.

And then you die.

SPRING

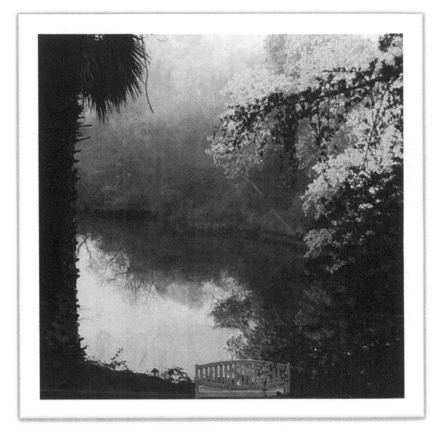

Napa, California

"This spring wakes us, nurtures us, revitalizes us.
"How often does your spring come?"
—Gary Zukav

"Never yet was a springtime,
when the buds forgot to bloom."
—Margaret Elizabeth Sangster

"Despite the forecast, live like it's spring."
—Lily Pulitzer

When the seasons change, so can we. It's true for every season, but it's especially true in spring, when all things blossom and grow. You can spring forward by focusing on the positive, setting goals, sticking with your plan, and nicest of all, being kind to yourself and others, including the annoying, unsupportive others. For many years, I've been training myself to eat more slowly, chew more consciously. It's a battle; I'm still the first one finished. I'm a work in progress, I tell myself. Some day, if it's important to me, I'll chew with more awareness. It's not that big a deal. All is well.

Spring Forward.

"Springtime is in the air," writes Kenneth Cohen, a Qigong master of the Tao. "A good time for spring cleaning of mind and body through meditation, healing practices, eating spring greens, drinking herbal tonics, and bathing in natural hot springs."

Before I shower you with my own suggestions about how to celebrate spring, let me ask: What's your number one wish when it comes to living a healthier life?

Think for a minute. We're not in a rush.

The truth is, we humans can make positive change any day—if we're really ready. But in spring, Mother Nature gives us an extra cellular push. Spring is the time of new beginnings, new growth. In spring, when all things made of light turn towards the light, it's easier for you to do the same.

Consider these five ways to get your sap rising:

Do something you're afraid to do. Fear can keep us from being the person we'd like to become. Over the next few weeks and months, face a fear...and work through it.

Volunteer at a hospice. Stop coloring your hair. Jump out of a plane, with an instructor, tandem, screaming.

When we overcome a fear, our whole body relaxes into a feeling of confidence and well-being. If I can do the thing I feared, what else can I do?

Look into your biochemistry. Face the facts. Most doctors know next to nothing about nutrition. It's lack of training more than lack of interest, I hope, but it means you have to make the effort yourself to figure out what foods, vitamins and supplements you need. Your nutritional profile—your biochemistry—is uniquely your own. Just because your best friend takes iron or vitamin B-12 shots, doesn't mean you should. The best strategy is to have basic blood work done and find a nutritionist who will analyze the results to determine what you personally need—and what you don't. Remember: Real food—unprocessed, locally grown, mostly organic—is the smartest way to get what your body needs. Supplements are always second, and they should only be taken as necessary, not because they are being promoted by your health food store.

Step up your physical activity. Most people insist they'd like to exercise more—more walking! more biking!—but when push comes to shove, they claim they don't have the time. Horse feathers. In reality, you *make* the time. You organize your day so there is time. This spring, stop making excuses and start organizing. If it means fewer hours on social media, congratulations.

A few more ideas spring to mind: Get up an hour earlier—to walk, to do yoga, to move your body in ways that feel good. Take the stairs instead of elevators and escalators. Keep a sturdy stationery bike next to the TV and sprint your way through every dopey commercial that pushes drugs you probably shouldn't ask your doctor about.

This spring, no matter how many times you've failed to make physical activity a priority, begin again. Plan for success, and celebrate in the summer with something you really want, like a new kayak or a standup desk.

Find your stress and let it go. Stress happens. It's unavoidable in this complex, anxious world. How you meet it and treat it is up to you, and that's worth working on this spring.

Choose an activity that heightens awareness and lowers your anxiety: Meditation? Cooking? Standup yoga on paddleboards?

Health experts agree that more than 75 percent of all sickness and disease is related to stress, in your body, and in your mind. That's an astonishing number.

This spring, find it in your body, and let it go. It's a little like throwing up –you'll know when it's happening.

Eat smart. Turn over a new leaf this spring—preferably spinach, kale or arugula—and swear off processed foods. Give your kitchen a spring cleaning—a mindful makeover. Read labels. If the so-called food has line after line of ingredients you can't pronounce, toss it. Don't continue to eat it or feed it to your children. And sugar? Cut back, cut down, and keep eliminating it, one donut at a time. If you wean yourself off sugar this spring, you'll sail through summer with a lightness you've never known before.

ENERGY EXPRESS-O!   Your Season to Blossom

"All beings are flowers
blossoming
in a blossoming universe."
—Soen Nakagawa

GOING DEEPER

Buy a notebook and write down the change you want to see for yourself this spring.

Why is this change important to you?

How will you make it happen?

Write down the details of your practice and keep track of your progress, focusing on the positive every step of the way. If you slip slide away for a day or a week, accept it, appreciate your rebellious nature, and get back to your journal. Journaling is to healthy lifestyle what wheels are to a car. It makes movement easier. It's also a time-honored way to focus your energy and attention so you can reflect on how things are going.

If you keep your journal in one place you visit every day—next to your toothbrush, under your keys—you are a thousand times more likely to write in it.

Maybe keeping a journal won't work for you. But maybe it will. It did for me. I was a junior size 15-16 when I graduated high school. My first journal was my path to changing the way I ate, and your journal can steer you in the direction you decide to go, keeping track to stay on track.

What do you have to lose?

Fear is nature's way of helping us grow. Fear holds us back from doing lots of stuff, until we overcome fear, and then we realize what a friend and ally it is. When I was young, I feared I'd never get over my stutter. How long will I b-b-b-b-be like this? How can I t-t-t talk in class? Marry a guy named P-P-P-Preston!? Over time, my stutter went away. Other fears followed—I used to go crazy when I'd see a spider—but now I have a point of view. And when I take that point of view on vacation, well, it leads to unforgettable experiences.

Make Your Getaway.

I've been a cheerleader for adventure travel since the first time I jumped on my bicycle and yelled, "Giddyup!" What's ahead, around the corner, up the trail? Who will I meet? What will I see? Why am I here?

My curiosity about the unexplored and unpredictable has led me to trekking in Tibet, kayaking down the Wisconsin River, hiking in the Rockies and hut-to-hut cross-country skiing in Vermont. (After only two lessons. Oye.)

Recently, I set a course I'd never been on before: sailing.

I'm actually a bit afraid of the sea. (It's wet, and there are all those unseen creatures!) But that didn't stop me from saving up and signing on for seven nights of sailing with friends in the small Cycladic islands of the Aegean, all doing our charter best to help Greece out of a devastating economic crisis she does not deserve.

Adventure travel, on the other hand, is something we all deserve. It's fun. It's challenging. It's mystical enough to teach you lessons you need to learn, and it has the potential to change your life in ways that five days at Disney World just can't.

Where you go isn't as important as planning an adventure that calls to you—whatever, wherever, whenever. You're never too old to be brave. All you need is the willingness to step out of your comfort zone and, in this case, onto the deck of a sweet 50-year-old 56-foot ketch with three cozy guest cabins and a magnificent and joyful master captain willing to take us wherever the wind and our seasickness would allow. (www.holidays-sailing.com)

Sailing is a sport. I wasn't sure it was before my week at sea, but now I know for sure: Sailing is work, physically and mentally. Whereas watching *other* people sail is a perpetual dream. There are mainsails and jibs to be raised, lines to be pulled, anchors to be set.

And more than brute strength and a strong back, you need focus. Total focus and intense concentration—and that's just for walking around the deck. Sailboats are loaded with lines, pulleys, fairleads and steel rigging tracks that sit there, waiting to snag any passing toe that isn't paying attention.

All of which led me to one of the great lessons learned on board, a teaching I keep hurrying back to: Slow down; take your time; stay in the moment. And get ice on that toe ASAP.

Pack light. Adventure travel requires you to lay out the stuff you need for the trip, and then leave half of it at home. Sailboats are all about storage, and the lack of it, so you have to make do with less. And having a strict sense of order will give you extra room to store more goodies, like potato chips and Greek butter cookies.

I know it sounds shallow, but one of the things I loved most about my first sailing journey was discovering I could wear the same shorts and T-shirt day after day and nobody cared, least of all me. I had that liberating insight on the tiny island of Despotiko, walking around the spectacular ruins of a 2,500-year-old temple of Apollo and Artemis, and by golly, I thanked them.

Stay active. Sailing involves a lot of sitting. Sitting and reading; sitting and eating; sitting and staring at clouds that suddenly take on the shape of Mrs. Blum, my seventh-grade math teacher. All worthwhile activities, but thank Neptune I brought my yoga mat. Swim, stretch, float...just don't sit, sit, sit. Find ways to keep your body juiced and open and your mind will follow.

Go with the flow. In nature, there is a divinely natural tendency to feel very small and very large at the same time. Being at sea, under the stars, brings wave after wave of realization that you are a tiny speck in an incomprehensibly deep universe, so there's no point in being anything but grateful for the life you have.

ENERGY EXPRESS-O!   To Sail Is to Surrender

"That's what sailing is, a dance, and your partner is the sea. ... She's the leader, not you. You and your boat are dancing to her tune."
—Michael Morpurgo

ENERGY EXPRESS

GOING DEEPER

The best way to discover the life-changing nature of adventure travel is to plan your own getaway.

What will it be?

Time on a trail with a horse—or a llama? A week of canoeing and camping out of Ely, Minnesota? Taking the bus to a nearby town and hiking home?

Where do you want to go—inside and outside—to break through your ordinary experience of life and allow an extraordinary experience to unfold?

You're in charge. You do the research. You decide. If you want others involved—as I always do—then make it a merry event, but stay close to your intention.

You don't have to go to Tibet to have a transformation.

An awakening can happen anywhere, anytime, to anyone. But it's more likely to happen in nature, when you're connected to the water, the trees and clouds, to the blue sky, to a felt sense of peace. All is well.

Now I have a miraculous little garden, but for years, I could only relish the possibility. I loved to listen to people who watered their curly endive and ate their own arugula and grew sweet basil on their back porch. "It's my meditation," one friend confided, and I swooned with a bad case of greens envy. And flowers! What's more beautiful than a vase filled with saucer sized tulips from your own yard? But beware. Gardening can be a source of pain if you don't know beans about preventing injuries. Your most personal fitness trainer offers up a short-course on growing your awareness.

Dig Into Nature.

Are you into gardening? Please say yes. Food you grow yourself tastes better, costs less, has greater nutritional value AND it leaves a carbon footprint the size of a grape. It's a kind of miracle. I can't think of a mean thing to say about it, except...

Gardening isn't an aerobic sport, and it won't grow your fitness the way running, walking, and biking will. But it sure can produce lots of pleasure, not to mention Green Goddess cauliflower, Box Car Willie tomatoes and Purple Passion asparagus.

Gardening also helps you cultivate a calm, focused mind while you're putting all the major muscles of your body to work—digging, lifting, and carrying. Besides burning calories, gardening connects us to the earth, and it's that mindful exchange of energy—you plant, nature grows—that is so joyful and satisfying.

Growing stuff in a garden is also a splendid way to plant ideas in your child's brain about what real food is, and how good it can taste. Next thing you know, your 10-year-old is snacking on kale chips instead of corn chips, and he goes to sleep at night dreaming of broccoli stalks the size of baseball bats.

Well, not immediately, but over time. Tending to a little garden—even a flowerpot on the windowsill—can give your child a wondrous sense of being connected to nature. It's a good thing.

Gardening is right up there with fly-fishing as a low-injury activity. But you still need awareness. If you rush into your garden chores carelessly, tweeting and texting, your mind a million miles away, you can wrench your back, create crippling tension in your shoulders or wind up with a neck stiffer than a newborn zucchini.

So before you start growing a list of gardening aches and pains, consider the following:

Learn to lift and carry. Prepare before you lift. Take a breath or two and make sure your body is aligned and ready. Relax your head and neck, drop your shoulders, and ,when you lift, engage your core muscles (your abs, glutes, torso muscles on both sides of your spine, front and back.) Lift slowly, pushing down through your feet, and drawing up through your legs. No grabbing and snatching, and no undue pressure or strain on your lower back.

Carry heavy items (bags of fertilizers, rocks, prize-winning watermelons) close to your body, not out in front of you, arms outstretched. Give thanks for the wheelbarrow, and use one whenever you feel like it.

And finally, think it through before you do. If you think something is too heavy to lift or carry by yourself, it probably is. Macho is not an evolved state. Get help, and avoid a nasty injury.

Small bites avoid big problems. When you shovel or dig, be content to take small bites with good tools that fit your hand. Good gloves will protect those hands so find a pair you like, even if they're pink.

And just like in the gym, don't overdo it. Big shovels loaded with heavy dirt can easily strain your back, shoulders, and knees.

To avoid post-planting strains and sprains, keep your mind focused on the task at hand: smaller loads, no sudden twisting or torqueing, moving with awareness so you stay balanced and aligned.

A little protection goes a long way. Start with your knees. Protect their delicate structure by kneeling on a foam pad or towels. Protect your eyes with sunglasses and a hat. Protect your skin from the burning sun with a proper cover-up—clothes or nontoxic sunscreen—and by moderating exposure.

Begin your gardening with a little warmup, simple range-of-motion stretches that juice up your joints and energize your muscles for the work ahead. If you feel pain when you garden, back off, relax, and, if you start up again, look for an easier way to do the same task. Drink enough water to stay hydrated, and don't stay in any position too long.

Cultivate calmness. To make all your gardening chores more effortless, move with the flow of your breath. This can work wonders in all your activities, from shooting baskets to unloading your car. Focusing on your breath gets you started, but then it's up to you to immerse yourself in the moment and not distract yourself with memories of the past or worries for the future.

Growth sustains life. What's good for the plants is good for you, too. Once that seed is planted, you'll never want to buy another plastic box of tasteless tomatoes again.

ENERGY EXPRESS-O!   Peas and Prosperity

"Everything that slows us down and forces patience, everything that sets us back into the slow circles of nature, is a help. Gardening is an instrument of grace."
—May Sarton

GOING DEEPER

This week, do something related to growing food.

If you don't have room for a garden, plant a window box and fill it with the herb of your choice. Parsley, mint, basil, and rosemary will give you a taste of success with very little effort. And your dinner guests will go crazy when they see you showering their plates with chopped homegrown parsley.

If you don't have space for a window box, join a community garden.

Or ask a friend with outdoor space if you can take a bit of it to grow some tasty greens or other stuff you'd like to share.

The ultimate goal is to get your hands in the soil and wiggle them around.

Wiggle your nose around, too. Inhale and exhale deeply, until you know what the earth smells like.

Compound that feeling with gratitude…and your spirit will grow faster than a radish.

Do you have too much stuff? It's a privilege...and a curse. More stuff—more clothes, more electronics, more storage containers in more colors, more, more, more— doesn't bring you more happiness. It leads to physical clutter and mental muddle, and both wear down our sense of well-being, not to mention our prefrontal cortex. Take it from me, owner of way too many T-shirts, including one from Chicago's first marathon in 1976, the same year I started to run with my fitness column. Some day, I keep telling myself, I'll choose 35 and do a quilt.

Sort Yourself Out.

Remember last December 31? It was the night you popped the champagne, screamed "enough!" and resolved to do something positively healthy in the new year.

Learn to cook! Lose 30 pounds! Get to the gym three times a week! Stop after one glass! (OK, two.) Find time to meditate 10 minutes a day, *no matter what!*

Proclaiming our best intentions is a piece of cake compared to sticking with them. Be honest: Have you seen a real change in yourself these last couple of months?

Don't worry. I've had cheeses last longer than many of my year-end resolutions. "Insanity," Albert Einstein told us, "is doing the same thing over and over again and expecting different results."

Dear reader, you may have tried some of my favorite action steps: Write down your goals, make them small and achievable, and keep a journal of your progress. But if you've failed time and again to make lifestyle change happen, and you want a *different* result, try doing something different, even if it strikes you as wacky and woo-woo.

I'm proposing that you clear the space. According to the time-honored principles of feng shui—much ridiculed, highly respected—clutter in your home and in your workspace can be a real block to change. The same is true of your mind. When you clear the space—physical and mental—magic can happen.

Christan Hummel is a pro at this. Here are a few of her best ideas, taken from her classic "Do-It-Yourself Space Clearing Kit."

Respect your space. Energy follows thought, says Hummel. So don't bring bad energy into your home. Take off your shoes and leave them at the front door as a way to consciously let go of your concerns of the day. That was before. This is now. Now, in your home, you can shift to a more positive state. (Eastern philosophers have been teaching this for about a million years.)

Clean out bad energy. It's a subtle thing, but it just feels better to be in a personal space that is orderly and organized. Get ready to spring clean your closet, home, garage, both physically and energetically, by using essential oils like sage, smudging or even sacred sounds. Sage? Smudging? Bells and chimes? Yep, the most effective space clearing goes way beyond Spic 'n' Span.

Practice letting go. Make room for the new by consciously letting go of the old, on a deeply personal level. To mark the beginning of the rest of your life, perform a ritual, *do something different*. A classic way to mark the moment is to light a candle, write down what no longer serves you— from addictions to anger—and feed it to the flame, taking care not to burn down the house.

Get rid of stuff. Your home has a circulation system, says Hummel, and when you've got too many possessions gunking it up, the energy you need to make change cannot flow. Recycle, give, or throw stuff away. Practice "emotional release work." That's when you privately honor, love, and appreciate the item (and the person who gave it to you) just before kissing it goodbye.

Another champion of sacred decluttering is Marie Kondo, the best-selling author of "The Life Changing Magic of Tidying Up." Her popular book truly can be life-changing if you're willing to follow her KonMari method of transforming your messy spaces (and messy life) into "spaces of serenity and inspiration."

"My clients never go back to the mess," she said in one of her wildly popular YouTube videos. "Once you find out what objects inspire you, you find out what inspires your life."

"Tidy up in one shot," Marie Kondo advises, "as quickly, and completely, as possible." And don't go room by room. She insists you go by category, not by location—all your clothes first, all your personal momentos last, because the more you do it, the easier it gets.

"Make sure you touch each thing," says Kondo. Then listen to your body. If the item sparks joy, keep it. If it doesn't inspire you, thank it for all that it has done for you, and let it go.

ENERGY EXPRESS-O! Does That Chipped Vase Spark Joy?

"Keep only those things that speak to your heart. …
By doing this you can reset your life and embark on a
new lifestyle."
—Marie Kondo

GOING DEEPER

If you think organizing your closets feels good, wait until you experience the pleasure and peacefulness that comes from organizing your mind.

That's the premise of a fascinating book called "Organize Your Mind, Organize Your Life: Train Your Brain to Get More Done in Less Time," by Margaret Moore, CEO of Wellcoaches, and Paul Hammerness, a Harvard Medical School psychiatrist.

Modern life is so demanding, we forget to focus. Left to our own devices, mostly digital, our prefrontal cortex is easily overwhelmed, leaving many of us feeling frenzied, distracted, and disorganized.

"It's an epidemic!" writes Moore, just like chronic multitasking, but the good news is you can train your brain to attain a higher sense of order and along with it, a sense of calm, wisdom, positivity.

How exactly? "Sleep well, exercise, do a mindfulness practice or choose the slow lane from time to time, even for a few minutes," writes Coach Meg, just hinting at a few of the learnable skills she and Hammerness discuss in their book.

When you organize your closet, you end up with extra hangers. When you organize your mind, you clear it of useless hangers-on and set yourself up for success in all realms.

Our bodies were meant to play and have fun. That's why denying kids recess in schools is such a cruel and stupid thing to do. Every body thrives when it meets the movement it loves to do. It could be softball or soccer, tango or trampoline, basketball or bocce ball. If you adore what you do, it's not work. And when you're in synch with your sport, it's not exercise. It's liberation! You are free to find joy in movement for the rest of your life.

Find Your Sport.

I've always believed there's a sport for everyone. Find it, and you're home free when it comes to living an active lifestyle. Years ago, I wiggled my way into race walking, an Olympic sport unknown to me before I went to a local spa for a few days of sun and silliness with some girlfriends.

It just so happened that Olympic champion race walker Augie Hirt was giving a workshop that weekend. It changed my life. Before Augie, I was a runner—a slow, lumbering, back-of-the-pack runner. When I discovered his sport, I found mine.

As a runner, I felt like a buffalo. When I race walk, I feel like a jaguar—sleek, nimble, vibrant. I love the hip wiggle, the heel strike, the way you straighten your front leg as you stride forward, twisting your torso from side to side. Yes, it looks goofy. So what? Ever watched snowshoe baseball?

"Wear a hat," I tell friends I've taught to race walk, "and sunglasses."

Is it better than running? I think so, but you can't tell that to a runner. Race walking works your lower body *and* your upper body, and it doesn't pound your knee joints the way running does. It also works miracles on the back of your thighs where cottage cheese tends to accumulate.

I can't teach you how to race walk writing about it— it's best to learn and practice with a human guide—but I do want to tell you some things you can do to take your own walking program to a higher, more athletic level:

Shorter, faster. Any style of walking is OK when you're just getting started, but there comes a time when you need to add some zip to your step. So that means taking longer strides, right? Wrong. Take shorter, quicker ones. That's the way to go faster.

Keep your head up. This small change will make a big difference. Walking with your eyes and head down is a common mistake. It strains your back and shoulder muscles, and you'll tire out quickly because it hinders efficient breathing. You are remembering to breathe, aren't you?

Move your arms. You'll be surprised how much more powerful your stride gets once you bring your arms into play. Don't hunch your shoulders or tense your arms. Allow them to swing in a relaxed and natural way, without crossing your midline in front. Keep your elbows tucked into your sides, arms bent at about a 90-degree angle. Don't clench your fists. Keep your hands loose. Feel and move like an athlete.

Work those hips. Someday you may want to find your own Augie Hirt-style coach and learn the official race walking technique, including one foot on the ground at all times. Meanwhile, for power walking, allow your hips to extend forward with each stride. As your right leg comes forward, so should your right hipbone, in a natural rotation. Then your left. Race walkers get a lot of speed, forward thrust, and funny looks from this exaggerated hip wiggle. It takes practice and patience, but once you get it, it's yours forever.

Engage your glutes. As you walk, practice somatics. Be aware of engaging your abdominal muscles and your glutes. Think about urging them forward under your hips, causing a bit of a pelvic tilt. Walking this way—head up, stomach pulled in, glutes engaged—is a fantastic way to help tighten those areas that tend to get loose and flabby as we age.

Go for the roll. There's no wrong way to walk, but the right way, for maximum efficiency and power, involves walking heel-ball-toe. Focus on landing on your heel, your toes flexed to the sky, and then roll through the foot, using the big toe to give your body a powerful push forward. That way all your leg muscles are awake and involved. Walking this way makes for a better workout, but don't overdo it. Increase your time and intensity gradually, or your shins may start to talk back to you.

So please, dear reader, find your own sport—or grab your hat and sunglasses and try mine. You'll find everything you need to get started at racewalking.org and the YouTube race walking videos are good, too.

ENERGY EXPRESS-O! I'm Just Saying...

"If God had wanted people to run, he wouldn't have invented race walking."
—Rick Williams

GOING DEEPER

This is a no-brainer.

Search the internet for a race walking coach or club in your town.

Yes, it's possible to learn from videos, but I still believe it's best to learn from another human being.

Your job is to find that person. If they charge and it's not in the budget, beg a friend to share a beginner's lesson with you.

Once you get the hang of it, not to mention the wiggle, you can practice on your own for the rest of your life. And don't forget your hat.

No one is paying me to say this (darn!): The Varidesk changed my life. It's a standing desk that fits on top of my weathered wooden desk, and I wish everyone in the world would use some version of it. Here's why: Chronic sitting makes you sick. Over time, it contributes to a list of diseases and ailments as long as your tibias and fibulas combined. Sitting too much shortens your life. I stand amazed, and so, I hope, will you.

Stand Up for Yourself.

Sit happens. Everyday, millions of Americans spend 8 to 14 hours on their behinds, sitting. I'm talking to you. Think about your day: You sit when you drive, watch TV, answer emails, eat breakfast, lunch, dinner, and snacks, read a book, play a video game, admire your cat. The truth is, we modern Americans sit so much that it passes for totally normal behavior. We don't even think about it, do we?

Well, start thinking! Pull up your life-shortening chair and listen to this: There are now over 10,000 studies showing that too much sitting is a terribly destructive thing to do to your health and well-being.

Rise to the truth. Your body thrives on movement, and when you make it sit for hours at a time, you create serious damage at a cellular level. Research shows prolonged sitting significantly raises your risk of developing heart disease, obesity, diabetes, cancer, insomnia, arthritis, osteoporosis. That's for starters. It's hard to believe chairs are still legal. If 70 is the new 50, sitting is the new smoking.

And don't think your daily workouts will protect you. Nope. Chronic sitting is an *independent* risk factor, meaning all the risk correlations hold true no matter how much you exercise. It sounds too bad to be true, *butt* it is.

And that's why I want to focus not on the sitting-kills research, (astonishing as it is) but on what can you do to sit less, micro move more and educate yourself about the benefits of standing:

Use a standing desk. If sitting kills, standing saves. That's why standup desks are quickly rising in popularity, in offices, in homes, and especially at *my* home, where I'm happily standing now, in front of my new Varidesk, a clever, affordable design in the $350 range that I've been showing off to friends like a new puppy.

Some standups I researched looked too corporate and would have meant replacing my beloved old wooden desk. The Varidesk sits on top and has an easy, spring-assisted lift that takes me from sitting to standing in a couple of seconds. I love it…and I'm pretty sure it loves me.

It comes with an app for standup alerts, but I'm just using my own body awareness—gradually standing longer and longer until my legs tire, and then sitting for 30 minutes or so before I rise again.

I found a ton of anecdotal evidence online about standup desks curing back pain, insomnia, fatigue and more, and I'm not surprised. But too much standing can also create health problems (varicose veins, for instance) so stay tuned into your body and rest in your chair when you need to.

Move more. One sure cure for too much sitting is getting up every hour and moving for 10 minutes or so. Is that so hard? Apparently, yes. So do what you have to do— an app, a phone alert, a kitchen timer—to remind yourself to stand, to stretch, to do neck rolls, air squats, and other energizing movements. There's also walking to the water cooler, jumping rope, practicing your tango moves.

Mercola.com is an excellent source for videos demonstrating the kind of intermittent exercises you should be doing, standing up and moving at least once every hour. "I was able to reduce my normal 12 to 14 hours of sitting to under one hour," Dr. Joe Mercola reports. "And I noticed one amazing thing—the back pain I've struggled with for many years simply disappeared."

Read this book. If you want to understand the solid science behind standing, read Dr. James Levine's recent book, "Get Up! Why Your Chair Is Killing You and What You Can Do About It." He's the Mayo Clinic endocrinologist and pioneering researcher who documented the perils of too much sitting in 2000, way before it was accepted as true. And now he's a leading voice for change in the work place, at home, and very importantly, in schools, where prolonged sitting hurts kids and stifles creativity.

I hope you're convinced. Stand more; sit less! Now it's time for me to lower my desk and rest my...case.

ENERGY EXPRESS-O! Rise Up to Change Course

"Sitting is more dangerous than smoking, kills more people than HIV and is more treacherous than parachuting. We are sitting ourselves to death."
—James Levine

GOING DEEPER

To get the feel of a standing desk, rig up something at home using books or a box. Ideally, you want the screen of your computer at eye level and your hands on the keyboard at a 90-degree angle. You might want to invest in a wireless keyboard to get the proportions right, but before you do, experiment with the best set-up you can.

Don't be frozen in your standing position. Unlock your knees, bounce up and down on your toes a few times, let your hips sway from side to side, pump your pelvis gently, curling and uncurling your tail bone.

Small, nourishing movements energize your body.

Just use your common sense, and don't overdo it.

And when you feel tired, dear reader, please be seated. Too much standing can leave you with sore legs and aching hips, neither of which is fun or necessary. As your body adjusts and gets stronger, you'll find yourself standing longer and longer.

It's great for the core!

I've made a lot of remarkable discoveries over the past 40 years, but nothing beats discovering the effect of making teeny-tiny movements inside your own body. These small somatic moves, a mix of science and art, enliven the subtle energies. Don't turn me in to the AMA, but I've successfully used somatics to relieve a painful shoulder, unblock a jammed knee, and otherwise infuriate many M.D. pals of mine who have no idea what I'm talking about. It's not foolproof, but what is?

Start Very Small.

When we humans imagine ourselves "exercising," we tend to focus on playing sports, working out in the gym, going for a 30-minute walk. Yes! All great ways to boost your energy and give your body the juiciness and joy it deserves.

But please don't limit your exercise routine to these big-picture pursuits. There is the outer game—played out on soccer fields, tennis courts, treadmills—but there's an inner game, too, going on inside every interconnected nerve, cell, muscle, and bone of your body.

And if you're not making *that* connection, you're missing out on a wonderful, almost magical, opportunity to improve your well-being.

Sense your sacrum. Let's focus on the sacrum, to begin to shift your thinking. Do you know precisely where yours is? You should. Your sacrum—the Greek word for sacred bone, where the old masters believed the soul resides—is holy ground when it comes to the health of your lower back, your legs, your everything. It is centrally located at the base of your spine and if it's not stable, strong, and in balance, it can pinch, bite, and break you, in the form of a back pain, leg pain, numbness, tingling, and worse.

The inner game begins as you connect to your skeletal-muscular self, using an anatomy book for guidance, or learning from an evolved teacher, or engaging with the detailed images at www.innerbody.com, where you can pilot through the body using 3-D rotating images.

So, zoom in on the sacrum, the large triangular shaped vertebrae that joins up with your hipbones to form your pelvis.

Admire the architecture, front and back, right and left side. Notice how it sits between the two pelvic crests (called the ilium). Now find your own sacrum. Frame your two hands around it. I like to relax my thumbs onto my pelvic bone and flip my fingers around so they are pointed toward my spine, resting on both sides of the sacrum. Hello, sacrum. How ya' hanging?

Anatomy is destiny. Between the sacrum and the ilium is the notorious sacroiliac joint, or SI joint. The SI joint—the star of many a yoga class—stabilizes your pelvis and lower spine whenever you do any kind of movement. See how important your sacral region is?

And here's another ain't-nature-grand fact. When you're young, your sacrum starts out as five individual bones, or vertebrae. During late adolescence, the five vertebrae begin to merge, and by the time most of us are 30 years old, our sacrum has formed into one single bone, roughly the size of your hand.

Your sacrum is a very strong bone, because it has to be. Besides protecting all the spinal nerves of the lower back, and the entire female reproductive system, the sacrum supports the weight of the upper body as it spreads across the pelvis, into the legs. It also locks the hipbones together on the back and supports the base of the spinal column as it interacts with the pelvis. The bone itself has a spongy interior, and it appreciates nourishing fluids.

A happy sacrum is a balanced sacrum. Once you focus on the architecture of your sacrum—complex, connected—you'll understand why having a sense of it makes sense.

How does your sacrum feel when you bend forward from the waist slowly? Or arch your back? Is there tightness? Imbalance? Are there twinges? Self-care begins when you sense and listen to your body, to the clues it is giving you about how it feels, what it needs.

And what it needs in the sacral region is stability, strength, and enough juice to keep the nerves that pass through the sacrum moist and happy.

Which brings us back to exercise, and the science of going small, with somatics training, yoga, Qigong, the Alexander Technique, Pilates, Feldenkrais and more.

Even the best doctors were flat-out wrong when they used to tell people with lower-back pain to go to bed and rest their back until it got better. The opposite is true. Now doctors will tell you that it's slow, subtle, gentle exercise that helps ease the pain and promotes healing.

They know better now, and so do you. Start small.

ENERGY EXPRESS-O! The Body Is Amazing

"This new mode of functioning awakens us to the amazing self-sensing, self-organizing, and self-renewing system that we are."
—Risa F. Kaparo

GOING DEEPER

There's nothing like reading a good book.

Unless it's reading three very good books, all about somatics.

A new one, thoughtful and compelling, is by my friend, Tias Little, a master yoga teacher. It's called "Yoga of the Subtle Body: A Guide to the Physical and Energetic Anatomy of Yoga," an elegant book steeped in poetry and metaphor, not to mention anatomy, physiology, and neuroscience.

"Somatics: Reawakening the Mind's Control of Movement, Flexibility and Health" is the groundbreaking classic by Thomas Hanna. Motor sensory awareness is his thing, and his five-minute daily program is one that can help almost anyone "maintain the pleasures of a supple, healthy body."

Another inspiring and innovative work I've lugged around for ages is "Awakening Somatic Intelligence: The Art and Practice of Embodied Mindfulness" by psychotherapist Risa Kaparo, Ph.D. It incorporates mindfulness, visualization, breathing exercises, postures, and stretches into one big life-changing whole.

Pick one. Read it. Discover why making the mind-body connection is such a useful tool to have in your healthy lifestyle box, unlike, let's say, chemical-laden commercial sunscreens.

One reason I adore yin yoga is wrapped up in this teaching: "You don't use your body to find the pose, you use the pose to find your body." Yes! When you link to your body, slowly, through your breath, you can go deeper into your pose, your sport, your everyday experience of life. Float your kidneys. Lengthen your tailbone. Open the wings of your lungs. Is that even possible, you might ask? Is my tailbone really longer? I promise you, it doesn't matter.

Think in Pictures.

Feeling stressed? Oh, yeah. It's part of being alive. The tight shoulders, the sore neck, the nagging ache that slips down your spine until it gets to your lower back and locks you in pain. We've all been there.

Which is why I want to introduce you to yin yoga. It's unique characteristic is long, three-to-five minute holds, combined with subtle pumps, slow stretches, conscious breathing, and eye-opening visualizations. You begin to think in pictures.

This ancient practice is the pause that truly refreshes. It's about as far from situps and pushups as kite surfing is from floating in a pool with a mojito in your hand.

And here's the part you must believe: Yin yoga is accessible to all, even if you don't know a tree pose from a tree frog.

I took two yin yoga classes last week—in my family, we call this research—and at some point, as my constricted chest opened and I imagined warm honey pouring out of my heart, I had a revelation. This little-known form of yoga—this blissful experience of letting go and creating flow—is a wonderful way to become more flexible, less stuck. And it's so easy. If only people knew!

So let's begin. In all of yoga, you start where you are, but with yin yoga, it's especially true. It's a class in deep release and relaxation, what some teachers call restorative yoga. But yin yoga has its own special twist.

For one thing, it moves very slowly. In an hour or so, you might only get to five or six different postures. Be grateful for these long holds. It's a wonderful way, perhaps the only way, to release the bands of connective tissue that only get tighter and more restrictive as we age, as we sit, as we move too quickly through life. (You talking to me?)

Most exercise we do—running, biking, dynamic forms of yoga like ashtanga—is considered yang. In simplest Taoist terms, yang is the expansion force; yin is the contracting force. Yang exercise works on muscle through rhythm and repetition but does ziltch for your connective tissue. And that's what we humans want to access to have a more fluid and healthy body.

In a yin yoga class, you're given instruction, and permission, to mindfully explore and expand the tight connective tissue. Your breath is clearing the way—mentally and physically—for a healing flow of energy into and surrounding your hips, your knees, your spine.

The trick to loving your yin yoga class is learning what to do with yourself once you've eased into your posture. Five minutes can be boring, or it can be a journey of exploration, an active emptying.

First, you might give in to the tendency to look around the room to see who is holding their toes and who can't even see them. But I don't recommend it. Yoga is not a competitive sport. Someone is *always* more supple than you are. So what?

Second, instead of those sideway glances, direct your focus inside. Visualize the deepest part of your structure relaxing, expanding, letting go. Think in pictures. I repeat this, in case you already forgot.

Third, play with your breath. It's not a religious belief. It's a way of connecting your body to your mind, and the moment you try it you can feel the effect. When you go with the flow, your breath helps unblock and release, opening up and juicing up what is known in yoga as the subtle body.

There's nothing subtle about the benefits of yin yoga. So here are some highlights from a life-changing workshop I did with yin yoga master Paul Grilley some years ago in Chicago. He's been teaching since 1980, and his website is a wonderful resource for yin yoga information and study, including his revealing collection of bone photos.

Yin yoga stills, and then restarts, the flow of energy. Grilley teaches you that your connective tissue isn't just some inert gristle that keeps your knees in place and your back from going out.

Your connective tissue is a river of life-giving energy that flows through your entire body. It follows the meridian pathways described in the ancient texts on acupuncture, a flow of energy (also known as "chi") that can reach and nourish every cell and organ in your body.

Accept what is. Grilley began our workshop by pulling thighbones and pelvises out of a canvas bag and laying them on the floor. Talk about an attention getter. Structural limitation is real, says Grilley, pointing to all the shapes and sizes laid before us.

An anatomy expert, he wants you to understand that the unique angle and shape of your bones determines what you can do in yoga, no matter how many hours you spend willing your head to touch your toes.

"Your anatomy is yours! Your femur is different than the person next to you! All your good intentions and instruction—relax and let it open!—can't push you past your compression point."

Translation? You may never do the splits, or sit in full lotus, no matter how hard you push. That's OK, says Grilley. Focus your attention within the pose, not on how it looks, but how it feels.

"Yoga isn't about imitating a posture, it's about unblocking energy, moving your chi."

Chi whiz.

ENERGY EXPRESS-O!   Why We Practice

"Yoga is the perfect opportunity to be curious about who you are."
—Jason Crandell

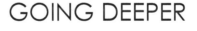

GOING DEEPER

Your curiosity is aroused. Can you really melt your connective tissue enough to touch your toes or release a tight lower back?

Find an experienced, inspired yin yoga teacher, and go at least three times, just to see if you want to stick with it.

Reread this column before every class.

If you find yin yoga boring, explore that sensation without giving it a name. Just witness yourself being bored.

As you engage in a little mind-body conversation—Is my sacrum level? What's that sensation in my hamstring?—you'll notice that your boredom is transformed into something else. You don't have to give that a name either. Just notice it.

Ideally, you'll entice a friend to experience some yin yoga classes with you. It's fun to have someone to talk to, to listen to, when class is over.

Misery loves company, but so does bliss.

It's too soon to know for absolutely certain what the Trump administration will do, if anything, to make our citizens healthier. Will they pay people to join a gym? Decide clean rivers are better than toxic rivers? Turn Michelle Obama's White House garden into a putting green? But here's one thing I know for sure: Our personal well-being ultimately depends on our own choices, much more than whom we have chosen to be president. What we eat and drink, how active we are, how much love we have in our life, and, yes, how happy we want to be.

Choose to Be Happy.

We are living in a Trumpian world. Personal well-being is under assault like never before. What will happen? The nail biting, world-changing election of Donald J. Trump as president of the United States is over, and this book is going to bed. What can a healthy lifestyle expert offer to inspire her readers?

Unconditional Happiness! It's one of my favorite classes at the University of Well-Being, Ballet, and Refrigeration because it's so controversial, so fascinating to consider, so essential if we are to remain strong and clear and move on with our lives in a way that promotes healing, defeats depression, and uncurls our toes.

Unconditional Happiness is the practice of choosing to be happy, no matter what. No matter who is lying, no matter who is resisting, no matter the state of our confused nation, you can lift your spirit and boost your health by answering this one question: "Do I want to be happy or do I want not to be happy?"

Michael Singer, an expert in Unconditional Happiness, calls it a simple question. But for most of us, it's impossibly complex. How can you be happy when your civil liberties are threatened, your spouse dies, your house disappears in a mud slide, your lover leaves you and takes the cat?

"Once you decide you want to be unconditionally happy, something inevitably will happen that challenges you," Singer explains in his New York Times best-seller, "The Untethered Soul."

Accept your life as it unfolds, Singer teaches. Don't let what happens make you miserable. If your answer to the "Do I want to be happy?" question is yes, then you have to let go of all conditions that arise. "You have to mean it regardless of what happens."

I told you it was controversial.

"When everything is going well, it's easy to be happy," writes Singer, who went from a penniless yogi to the founding CEO of a billion-dollar public company. "But the moment something difficult happens, it's not so easy.

"The question is not whether they will happen," Singer writes. "Things are going to happen. The real question is whether you want to be happy regardless of what happens. The purpose of your life is to enjoy and learn from your experiences. You were not put on Earth to suffer. You're not helping anybody by being miserable."

You can and should be vigilant, concerned, aware, involved in whatever distressing situation comes your way, Singer explains, but you can't let it get in the way of your commitment to be happy. Well, you can, but that's not the path to personal well-being.

"Committing yourself to unconditional happiness will teach you every single thing there is to learn about yourself, about others, about the nature of life," says Singer. "You will learn all about your mind, your heart, and your will. But you have to mean it when you say that you'll be happy for the rest of your life. Every time a part of you begins to get unhappy, let it go."

Easier said than done, it's true, but here's something else that's true.

"Regardless of your philosophical beliefs, the fact remains that you were born and you are going to die. During the time in between, you get to choose whether or not you want to enjoy the experience.

"Events don't determine whether or not you're going to be happy. They're just events. You determine whether or not you're going to be happy. You can be happy just to be alive. You can be happy having all these things happen to you, and then be happy to die."

Singer sets a high bar, especially for those who prefer going to a bar when something awful happens.

"If you want to be happy, you have to let go of the part of you that wants to create melodrama. This is the part that thinks there's a reason not to be happy. You have to transcend the personal, and as you do, you will naturally awaken to the higher aspects of your being."

That's when that overwhelming feeling of well-being kicks in, because you've made that strong choice.

"No matter what happens, just enjoy the life that comes to you," Singer says.

No matter what.

ENERGY EXPRESS-O!   Hungry for a Laugh?

"I'm not crazy about reality, but it's still the only place to get a decent meal."
—Groucho Marx

ENERGY EXPRESS

GOING DEEPER

The day after Donald Trump was elected president, author Jack Kornfield wrote: "When times are uncertain, difficult, fearful, full of change, they become the perfect place to deepen the practice of awakening."

Are you up for an awakening? That's at the heart of a healthy lifestyle, and so are these suggestions from Susan Piver, founder of the Open Heart Project:

Be generous. When we are afraid, we feel powerless. However, generosity is a gesture of power. So if you are feeling numb, aggressive, fearful, reach out and help someone else who is struggling. It's good for others, Piver says, and it's a very good thing to do for ourselves.

Remember that nothing is ever, ever as good as you hope or as bad as you fear. Take it one day at a time, Piver says. One day, one thought, one moment at a time. Meditation teaches you how to meet your experience on the spot, fully and courageously. Practice when you can.

Elect yourself president. "Your life—your home, family, friends, workplace, body, abilities—are your kingdom," writes Piver. You're the ruler in charge. What can you do for your world? Who or what needs your attention? Now is the time for you to remove every obstacle that stands in the way of doing your true work in the world. Please get on with it.

Express your love for your brothers and sisters.
Piver isn't suggesting that we get all snuggly with the
hatemongers, the racists, the anti-Semites, but she asks us to
acknowledge we are all Americans. This is our country.
United we stand, divided we get very, very nervous. Seeking
to excise 50 percent of our brothers and sisters from our
hearts and minds is not the higher path, and it extends
suffering.

Feel what you feel. Don't pretend you aren't scared,
sad, angry, and shocked, if you are. That's not a problem.
What is a problem is to avoid what you feel and take it out
on others by vilifying them. Terrible people must be held
accountable for terrible things. But grasping at aggression
keep us from seeing clearly the best course of action.

And what is the best course of action? Awaken.

When I was growing up—taught by my softball-loving dad to catch and throw 'like a boy'—girls were never encouraged to work with weights. "It's not feminine." "You'll bulk up." Crapola of all sorts. Strength training was for the guys, while the girls at South Shore High School earned gym credits for keeping their shoes chalked white and their hideous green gym suits starched and ironed. That was then. This is now. Now is about a million times better.

Play to Your Strength.

Summer is around the corner, and so are shorts, sleeveless tops, and swimsuits—all in bright colors and zippy designs that often reveal doughy arms and generous thighs.

A few rounds of golf can't help you. You can run a 10K every weekend, or hike, bike and play tennis till the cows come home ("who has cows?" you're asking), and *still* the most efficient way to build muscle and overall body strength is targeted strength training.

There are other good reasons for strength training beyond looking good in a bikini. Strong bodies are linked to strong minds. Strength training builds confidence, muscle and healthy tissue. It's also good for stable joints, injury prevention and weight loss. And yet—slugs that we are— fewer than 25 percent of Americans over the age of 45 work with weights on a regular basis. A whole lot fewer, I'm guessing.

Blame it on our sedentary lifestyles. The heaviest thing most of us lift is our laptop. Nothing we do requires us to raise our arms over our heads. Everyday chores may work the front body, but what about the back body, the side body, the subtle body inside your own body that benefits from a balanced program that builds muscle from top to bottom, back to front, side to side?

So for all those reasons and a superset more, here are eight strength-training truths to consider—as you decide how and when you'll get started:

There's no age limit. Little kids have to wait until their bodies and bones are strong enough to take the stresses of weight training, but the rest of us can start where we are, and can expect to see big improvements over time. The body is magnificent that way. People in their 90s are pumping iron and getting stronger, and so will you, once you understand the basics.

Technique is everything. This is a weighty matter, because if you don't learn to lift consciously, with awareness of your breath, posture, core, and limitations, you can strain a muscle or tear a tendon. Find an evolved teacher/trainer, or teach yourself from books or online videos.

Lift heavier weights. You won't get stronger lifting the same five- or ten-pound weight day after day, rep after rep. For your muscles to grow stronger, you need to challenge them—gradually, over time—with heavier weights. The "right" amount of weight will always vary, but this principle remains the same: You should be able to do ten or so reps with perfect form, with the last two being a real struggle.

Machines vs. free weights. Both will build strength. Using machines in a gym usually come with a price tag. Free weights speak for themselves: anytime, anywhere. Machines have a limited range of motion; free weights have infinite possibilities. *Both* can work if you work, intensely, consistently, thoughtfully, with proper attention paid to form and breathing. Body-weight exercises—squats, pushups, lunges—should also be part of your routine, which is why it's smart to consult with someone knowledgeable when you're first starting. (Lifting your body weight in yoga builds strength, too, but today I'm showing you how well-rounded I can be.)

Expect soreness. It's called DOMS—delayed onset muscle soreness—and it's what you can expect after a good workout. Pain is different. "No pain, no gain" is no way to approach a sustainable strength-training practice. If your trainer thinks otherwise, find one with a bigger brain.

Know your body. Spend a little time looking at anatomical drawings so you'll know your kidney from your colon, your patella from your pubic bone. Developing better body awareness will help you create and execute a balanced workout: front to back, side to side, pushing and pulling, expanding and contracting.

Be efficient. A 20-minute workout can be just as good as a 40-minute workout, if you know what you're doing and why. Compound movements, for example—a bicep curl combined with a lunge—will give you twice the benefit in half the time. So will super-slow lifting and high-intensity interval training. Again, study up and experiment until you find a routine that sparks joy. If you manage to do it two or three times a week, over time your body will change in remarkable ways, unless you celebrate every workout with two granola bars and three beers.

Use it or lose it. It's an inconvenient truth that as we age, we lose muscle and grow weak unless we make the effort to stay strong, flexible, agile, and juiced. It's about working with what you've got for as long as you've got, and being grateful in between.

ENERGY EXPRESS-O: The Reason We Train

"It is never too late to be what you might have been."
—George Eliot

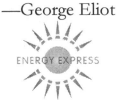

GOING DEEPER

If decide to lift weights, buy some time with a trainer who can teach you proper form and breathing.

These are learnable skills, and when you feel ready, you can drop the coaching and continue on your own.

But if you start off doing it wrong—holding your breath, jerking the weights, moving too quickly—you can create injuries, miseries, and doctor bills.

If you can't afford one-on-one time with a trainer, find a friend to share the cost.

Or take a strength-training class at a local Y or rec center.

Once you're set with the basics, you can set up a home practice space for $100 dollars or less, including a good yoga mat for proper stretching, warm up, cool down.

Don't wait! Begin your strength training this week. Your biceps will begin to take shape, and before you know it, muscle by muscle, week by week, you'll be defining a new you—buffer, bolder—and you'll be considering sleeveless tops.

Summer

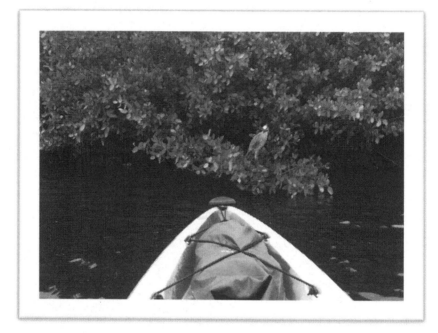

Robinson Preserve, Florida

"Summer afternoon—-summer afternoon; to me,
those have always been the two most beautiful
words in the English language."
—Henry James

"There's this magical sense of possibility that
stretches like a bridge between June and August. A
sense that anything can happen."
—Aimee Friedman

"Smell the sea, and feel the sky.
Let your soul and spirit fly."
—Van Morrison

I plan to grow up to be a magnificent elder. Look at the old lady in the punky haircut, they'll say, loved and loving at 93, still hiking, still laughing, still dancing till dawn (OK, midnight). A long life is part luck, part grace and— what else? I'd always wondered. And then I discovered the Blue Zones. The mystery of exceptional aging is no mystery at all. There are guidelines to be followed, insights to be shared, rules we can respect. One of my favorites involves waking up every morning with a passion and a purpose that gives your life meaning. When that ends, so will you.

Live Long, Die Happy.

This is the time of year I live, play and work on a tiny, remote Greek island with no airport and fewer than 3,000 residents, goats included.

It's a beautiful, magical, revelatory place. Be happy for me. A generous spirit is a sign that your healthy lifestyle training is paying off.

Of course, I take the World Wide Web with me, so anxiety is never far away. And neither is the island of Ikaria, one of the world famous Blue Zones, seven well-studied communities where surprisingly large numbers of people live into their 90s and beyond, and are vigorous, healthy, and relatively happy right to the end.

I can see Ikaria from my terrace, high above the Aegean, sipping a glass of cold retsina, chipping away at a chunk of freshly made feta cheese with wild oregano on top. It's a form of research. It inspires me to ask this age-old question:

Why do some people live so much longer than others?

Genetics play only a small part in longevity, 20 percent or less. Much more important are your personal lifestyle choices: What you eat and drink; the amount of physical activity you do; the time you spend with family and friends; how you handle tension, trauma, the ticking of the clock.

Ikaria—25 miles long, 5 miles wide, with healing hot springs that have made it a tourist attraction since 600 B.C.—has been studied up one mountainside and down the other. Blue Zone researchers want to determine what keeps Ikarians living so long, so well, with so little heart disease and diabetes, and virtually no dementia.

Let me repeat that last part before I forget: In Ikaria, dementia is practically unknown. In the U.S. dementia is rampant, costly, and incredibly scary.

In the U.S., only one in nine baby boomers will live to the age of 90, according to Dan Buettner, head of the Blue Zone movement. On Ikaria, one in three live to 90 and beyond.

Amazing. What do they know that we've forgotten?

You can find the answers in great detail at BlueZones.com. However, here's my summary, after spending some sweet days, walking and talking my way around Ikaria. I hope you're not too busy to read it:

Take your time. To live longer, slow down. On Ikaria, wristwatches are as useless as speed bumps. Ikarians are famous for moving at their own pace, working when they want to work, chilling when they want to chill. I learned that on my first visit there, having lunch with friends at a wonderful little taverna in the port of Agios Kirikos. We all ordered Greek salads. Some of us are still waiting.

Eat your greens. Over 150 kinds of wild greens grow all over the island, and Ikarians enjoy them in a variety of unusual salads and pies. It takes just the slightest bit of courage to stick your fork in. The island greens are a super source of antioxidants and are eaten, like almost everything else, with a splash of olive oil.

Drink herbal tea. Ikarians drink endless cups of tea made from wild mint, chamomile and other local herbs high in compounds that significantly lower blood pressure and decrease their risk of heart disease and dementia.

Take a nap. Ikarians take daily naps (about 30 minutes) at least five times a week. Blue Zone researchers calculate this lowers their risk of heart attacks by 35 percent! In a few of the mountain villages, they sleep by day and work and play through the night. Why? Because they want to.

(FYI: "Based on interviews," says Blue Zones expert Dan Buettner, "we have reason to believe that most Ikarians over 90 are sexually active.")

Keep moving. Many Ikarians live in mountain villages that require vigorous walking. They keep terraced gardens, tend to animals, and get lots of exercise every day without thinking about it.

Connect to community. Ikarians maintain strong social ties to their families, neighbors, and villages. They wake up feeling they have a purpose in life, whether it's tending to the great-grandchildren or feeding their chickens. They take time every day to meet face to face with friends, sipping Ouzo, shooting the breeze.

Eat the Ikarian way. Ikarians thrive on local fresh food, all of it organic and unprocessed. They avoid dairy but consume gallons of goat's milk, as yogurt or cheese. Their version of the gold-standard Mediterranean Diet is high in fruits and vegetables, beans, whole grains, potatoes, and olive oil. They drink a glass or two of local wine—absent nitrates and pesticides. (Some folks think it tastes like rotted leaf mulch; I like it. It could be a case of mind over matter.) And they benefit hugely from daily doses of their local honey, a thick amber-colored concoction rich in anti-bacterial and anti-inflammatory compounds.

Each of these Blue Zone guidelines could be a book. There is so much more to say, to do, to be. Maybe another time. You're free to go now. Time for a life-extending nap.

ENERGY EXPRESS-O! THE BLUE PEARL ZONE

"In the end, all that really matters is the state of your heart."
—Swami Chidvilasananda

GOING DEEPER

Choose one of the Blue Zone rules and plug it into your own life, no matter where you live or how old you are.

Slow down? More exercise? Guilt-free naps?

If you can't decide, try this one: Give yourself four olive-filled weeks on the Mediterranean Diet. I choke on the word diet, but in this case, it's come to mean a lifestyle choice, a super healthy way of eating that has nothing to do with denial and deprivation and everything to do with consuming real food, in moderate amounts, with a focus on fruits and vegetables, olive oil, whole grains, lean meats and fresh fish. There are many variations, but the core principals are the same, including a modest pour of red wine and enough time to slow down and savor every sip.

The Med Diet isn't for everyone. But in study after study, it keeps coming out on top as a way of eating that is good for all sorts of Westerners who want more energy, less bloat, and, over time, a comfortable, sustainable weight.

It's not about being thin. It's about eating real food, with real taste, and real advantages to your health and wellness.

If you come to love the Med Diet, and it becomes part of your lifestyle, bravo.

Next step? A week on Ikaria, possibly two.

I grew up loving sports. I wish I could say the same for French or algebra. Early on, my folks stepped up to the plate and made sure my sister and I knew how to ride a bike, hit a ball, swim, bowl, roller skate, jump rope, ride a horse and play tennis, golf, even horse shoes. It never mattered that we weren't the best. The message was: Have fun; learn something new; be a team player; don't break anything. I created "Energy Express," the Emmy-winning syndicated TV series about sports, fitness, and adventure, to inspire millions of kids to grow up loving to be active. It all begins when you're little.

Raise an Active Kid.

"Hit the ball! You're not concentrating!"

"Your baby brother could have caught that!"

"Run! Faster! You're not even trying!"

Lots of parents don't know how to behave when they watch their kid play sports. They're loud, and obnoxious, and super-critical. So how should they act? Differently.

Here are some vital parenting rules to help you lead your child into a life of active play, so they don't give up and drop out of sports before they've had a chance to find the one they love—as long as it's not football:

Be positive. If you can't say something nice during a game, say nothing at all. Or stay home. You're the parent, not the coach. Your job is to be supportive, encouraging, unconditionally loving. Keep your comments positive. Let go of the negative. Give your kid credit for showing up, for working well with her teammates, for being a good sport. These qualities are a thousand times more important to your kid's future well-being than the final score of the game.

Focus on fun. If you want your kids to relax and enjoy sports, you have to relax and enjoy watching. If you get upset and unruly, so will they. All the experts agree: The quickest way to kill a kid's interest in sports is to overemphasize winning. It's a game! The real victory is for your kid to feel comfortable and happy chasing a tennis ball or swinging a bat. Kids who are made to feel unworthy on the field take that insecurity into adulthood. It's not pretty.

Praise the effort in spite of the outcome. If your kid's team wins the game, bravo. But if your youngster is on the losing side, you need to offer empathy, not criticism. Recognize the loss, but don't dwell on it. The teachable moment is not about the value of winning but the value of resiliency. If you can develop that nothing-can-defeat-me spirit as a kid, being an adult gets a whole lot easier. Instead of dwelling on the loss, shift your kid's focus to something positive. Ask: What was the best part of the game?

Be available. Your behavior on game day is important, but a winning attitude at home counts, too. Do less talking and a lot more listening to your kid's experience. Don't judge. And don't box them in to playing soccer just because you grew up with posters of Pele in your room. Go join an adult soccer league and let your kids figure out what they love. Irish dancing? Trampoline? Cave diving? (God forbid.)

Stay above the fray. Sometimes fights erupt at a game, in the stands, on the field. Stay out of it. Don't abuse the refs or boo the other team. Stay cool, take a few calming breaths, and eat some apple slices till the argument blows over. It's also unwise to be critical of a coach in front of your kids. It you've got a question or complaint, take it up privately.

Keep your eye on the prize. Research shows that most kids play sports to have fun, improve their skills, and socialize with their friends. Winning isn't as big a deal to kids as it is to adults.

A much bigger deal is having your daughter or son feel good after the game. Fake praise won't do it. Kids are smarter than that.

If you parent with positive feedback and compassion when it comes to sports, your kid is much more likely to grow up enjoying an active, healthy lifestyle.

And that's the real goal, isn't it?

ENERGY EXPRESS-O! Try This on Your Kid Next Time

"We didn't lose the game. We just ran out of time."
—Vince Lombardi

GOING DEEPER

Plan a special play date with your own child, or one in your life.

Pick a sport neither of you have ever tried.

Cross-country skiing? Bird-watching? Ping-Pong?

Reread the "Raise An Active Kid" essay the night before you head out.

And again in the morning.

Remember that your goal, your objective, is to have a day of fun together.

Don't keep score. Keep laughing; keep smiling.

Win or lose, the goal is for both of you to end the day feeling like champions.

I know I'm a pain when it comes to promoting self-care. Someone shut me up. No one likes a nag. And yet, I can't resist: Your well-being is your responsibility. No one should be shamed or blamed for their health problems. Sickness happens. Diseases overwhelm us. We need skilled and compassionate health care workers to help us through. And yes, there are miracle drugs and miraculous surgeries that save lives. But in the end, it's your life, made up of your choices, big and small, healthy or not. Free will is even more powerful than free medical care.

Wake Up to Awareness.

Aches and pains are part of life. You wake up one morning and your back is tight, your shoulder is sore, your neck is jammed between two stone pillars. We usually accept these limitations and move on the best we can, with or without an Advil.

But here's the good news. Many of the aches and pains we live with or take painkillers for are caused by muscular imbalance. And muscular imbalance is often curable. By us, no prescription required.

Muscle imbalance is what happens when you use one set of muscles too much, and the opposing muscles a lot less.

It happens to everyone. You know what else happens? Costly visits to doctors. The overused muscles—over time—become inflamed and irritated. The underused muscles weaken and become vulnerable.

Once you realize how locked in you and your body are to repetitive patterns, you can begin to reprogram. It takes intense body awareness—also known as somatics training—which is probably why attention rhymes with prevention.

To prevent problems, you want to become aware of every day habits that create muscular imbalance, and for that, let's turn to a list compiled by fitness professional Beverly Hosford for the American Council on Exercise website:

Sleeping on the same side every night. If you always sleep on one side, or on your stomach with your head always turned the same way, switch sides. At first, it will feel odd. Explore that sensation. Remind yourself that you're on a path to a more balanced body. Then let go into dreamland.

Always leading with your dominant side when climbing. It's all about growing awareness. What foot leads going up stairs and what foot leads going down? Pay attention, and do what we're always doing in yoga to stay in muscular balance—switch to the opposite side.

Crossing your legs with the same leg on top. If you cross your knees or ankles when you sit, notice which leg sits on top. Do the old switcheroo.

Carrying bags on the same shoulder. Which shoulder do you normally use to carry stuff—groceries, kids, computer bags? Consciously shift your load to the other shoulder. What does *that* feel like? If you ever feel pain, stop. If you feel your shoulder is hunched and tense, release. Experiment with smaller loads, both sides.

Using the same hand to hold things. Which hand holds your phone, your fork, your toothbrush? Switch from time to time. This crossover trick is also good for your brain, breaking up old patterns, sparking new pathways. Will it feel weird? Will some toothpaste miss the mark?

Always putting your weight on one leg while standing. News flash! You're not an ostrich. So where is your weight when you're standing or leaning? To distribute the weight evenly, stand tall, your legs hip width apart, close your eyes. Shift your weight left and right, front to back, and settle into balanced, relaxed weight distribution from your feet to your head.

Locking your knees. Keep your knees soft when standing. Locking means you're blocking the flow of energy. Unlocked knees are happy knees, juicy knees, and when they're connected energetically to your feet, ankles, hips, and shoulders, alignment happens effortlessly. Relaxed and balanced muscles allow more energy to flow throughout your body. This is the "ready" stance for tai chi and Qigong, and it feels great.

Holding your phone or tablet at waist level. Text Neck is the next big thing in preventable, debilitating injuries. We all do it to see the screen—head down, neck scrunched, shoulders slouched—and we all will suffer the consequences...UNLESS we lift the screen to eye level (or use a device made to do this) and relax our neck and shoulders.

One-sided training in sports. For this one, just picture Rafael Nadal's forearm. Tennis, golf, and bowling are sports that obviously overdevelop one side of the body. Assess your sport for one-sidedness and correct the imbalance with focused weight training and cross-training, too.

Too much driving. Sit so your spine is aligned, your sacrum even, your shoulders relaxed. Take stretching breaks. Make tiny adjustments—mentally and physically—so your body is driving in a balanced, alert way.

That's it. It's all about bringing your body into balance, to working both sides, back to front, up one side and down the other.

It's up to you. It's your body, your responsibility to wake up and focus in.

Class dismissed, and as you walk away, please notice which leg is in the lead.

ENERGY EXPRESS-O! Keep the Faith

"If you think you are too small to make a difference, try sleeping with a mosquito."
—Dalai Lama

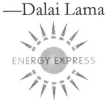

GOING DEEPER

The body is self-correcting, but first you have to notice.

So pick one everyday habit from the list above.

Ask yourself, because no one else will: Do I lock my knees? Stand with more weight on one foot? Carry bags on the same shoulder? Yes!

Awareness is first; taking action is second. Your gold star comes later.

That's the essence of self-care, and a requirement for being a lifelong mensch: When you see something that needs to be done, do it.

Lots of people think getting a relaxing, rejuvenating massage is a wild luxury. It's not. It's what self-care looks like. Sure it costs money, but so do addictive pain relievers and unnecessary surgeries. Why do most insurance companies pay for a $50 dollar box of Kleenex and refuse to reimburse you for a gifted body worker who releases stress, nourishes your muscles, and leaves you floating in a tub of butter? This pisses me off! But after a few minutes of deep pressure on the soles of my feet, all is well again.

Breathe In, Bliss Out.

I love a good massage. I even love a mediocre massage. I know there are people who can't stand being touched, and I respect that. But I also think they're nuts.

The older we get, the more we need wise and healing hands working us over, sensing our tight spots, stimulating blood flow, easing open the stuck places.

Sixty minutes is never enough. I'm an expert in healthy lifestyles. I believe in moderation, absolutely, but not when it comes to something as splendid for your body and mind and corporate demeanor as massage. It's like organic greens on your dinner plate—the more, the better.

Where do you hold tension? It's always a good idea to let your body worker know your personal preferences. I'm an absolute glutton for glute work. A mauled bun is a happy bun, free of tension, less likely to trigger lower back pain. Out, damned knot!

Massage equals prevention. In the best of all possible worlds, just now coming, massage therapy would be part of our regular maintenance routines, like having our teeth cleaned or our hairs cut.

Skilled body workers do things for us that need to be done, especially as we age. They relieve aching muscles, soothe joint pain, help prevent sports injuries and release energy blocks—physical and emotional—that keep us from living our healthiest, happiest life.

Many styles, many smiles. There is no one best massage technique. Massage is where the expression Different Strokes for Different Folks originated. Some of us like deep trigger-point work; others prefer lighter, longer strokes. And some like a sumo wrestler to dance on their spines.

No matter your choice—from hot stones to deep tissue, from Swedish to shiatsu—here are some suggestions that will make your next massage your best massage:

—Why lie there feeling guilty about the time or the money, when you could be congratulating yourself on your inner wisdom? Open up fully to the experience you are having. Stay in the moment, while listening to birds in a rainforest or some other soothing CD you were clever enough to bring along.

—Before your massage, scan your body for areas that feel tense or strained. Chronic soreness in your shoulder? Stiff neck? Tight quads? Tell your therapist, and then completely surrender to his or her touch. Engage your mind, and your breath, but let your therapist do the heavy lifting.

—Avoid idle conversation. Talking about a new movie or an old lover is a distraction for both of you. But, of course, give feedback when necessary, especially about the amount of pressure you want. The more still you are, the more you can tune in to the experience.

—Take a few deep breaths at the start to help you relax and get centered. If you begin to feel discomfort, don't clench or panic. Instead, exhale directly into the area of tension and visualize it melting away. If it works, great. If not, speak up (unless you're asleep). The best body workers will coach you to work with your breath during your session. Don't be shy about going with the flow, inhaling peace and joy, exhaling stress and credit card debt.

—A hot shower, bath or sauna can start the unwinding process before the massage. And your therapist will appreciate a clean body to work with.

—Don't come to the table with a full stomach. The less you have churning in your belly, the more comfortable you'll be. And remember to drink water afterward.

—Before you leave the session, ask your therapist to tell you about particular areas of tension or imbalance. (It could be your neck, your shoulders, your hips.) That feedback can help you pinpoint areas that you need to work on when you're off the table. I know I'm repeating, but hear me: It's these tight, tense, stuck places that contribute to injuries and illness later on.

Do-it-yourself massage works, too. If your budget is even tighter than your hamstrings, do what plenty of smart athletes do and learn to self-massage. Yoga, Qigong, and acupressure are splendid for that, and so is using a $25 dollar foam roller, with good form and thoughtful guidance.

Once a month? Once a week? Whenever I'm on the table—not thinking about the past, not thinking about the future—I'm thinking why don't I do this more? This is what self-care feels like. It's so much cheaper than a spinal fusion.

ENERGY EXPRESS-O!   Use the Force

"When the body gets working appropriately,
the force of gravity can flow through.
Then, spontaneously, the body heals itself."
—Ida Rolf

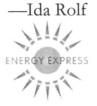

GOING DEEPER

I'll bet you think I'm going to suggest you book yourself a massage this week.

Wrong.

Instead, reach for the oil of choice and give someone you love your best version of a full-body massage.

If that sounds daunting, make it a foot rub.

Clear the space. Set the scene. Get in the mood and do what you can to get your partner in the mood, too. Music helps. So does dim light, no distractions, a total focus on what your fingers are touching, feeling, sensing as you massage his or her head, shoulders, back, legs, arms, hands, and don't forget the feet.If I've just lost you because your loved one would rise up, leave you, and move to Timbuktu if you tried anything like this this, then OK, book yourself a massage. Book ten.

The human touch. There's nothing like it. The technology of virtual reality is trying to take its place, but you can't beat the real thing.

And I don't mean Coke.

The number of people in America who live rock-solid sedentary lifestyles is heartbreakingly high. And mind-boggling, too. The human body is hardwired to move, to play, to frolic. That's how it thrives. That's how it grows. But I'm not panicking. Why? Because I'm 40 years into understanding the mechanics of self-sabotage, the way we create obstacles for ourselves, and what we can do—on our own, no prescription needed—to overcome them. We all self-sabotage, until one day, we don't. Today can be that day for you. And if it is, don't panic.

Resist the Dark Forces.

Is exercise good for you?

Duh.

Regular workouts give you strength, energy, a trimmer body, a healthier heart, a calmer mind and a much lower risk of at least 35 (!) different devastating diseases, including high blood pressure, stroke, osteoporosis, nonalcoholic fatty liver disease, diverticulitis, Type 2 diabetes, colon and breast cancer and, yes, even that star of prime-time TV: erectile dysfunction.

In spite of what we know, we don't do. According to the latest research, 92 percent of adolescents and 95 percent of adults in the U.S. do not meet the minimum guidelines for physical activity.

Oh, dear. When I think about the gap between what we know about the benefits of exercise vs. how much we actually do, my brain begins to sizzle.

And then I remember self-sabotage and the fire cools. Once you understand that there's a right way and a wrong way to approach exercise, your days as a self-saboteur are over.

Do it grudgingly, on remote control, impatient for quick results, and you are setting yourself up to fail. Do it consciously, finding pleasure, forgiving lapses, and your chances of lifelong success are greatly improved.

Here are some typical ways we humans sabotage own own fitness, and what to do instead:

You aren't truly committed. Saying you want to get in shape is not enough. You've got to have a deep-down, nothing-will-stop-me commitment. Change will happen only when you are ready, and when you are—halleluiah!—not only will you be able to overcome every obstacle; you will actually enjoy the process.

You have failed before. Many people don't understand that change is not linear. It's often two steps forward, one step back. Exercise dropouts have failed before, and the fear of failing again often makes them quit. You can break this self-defeating cycle by taking fear of failure off the table. See failure as feedback. Know you can succeed, and you will succeed, if you are patient and persistent.

You punish yourself instead of rewarding yourself. Negative self-talk will derail you. Listen to your inner voice. If it says you're lazy, stupid, ate too much and can't get to the gym today, tell it to take a hike. (Even a short one helps.) Start a new inner dialogue based on kindness and compassion for the healthier, happier person you want to be. Create positive affirmations, like "All is well," and repeat them often.

You compare yourself to others. Your best pal runs half-marathons and you struggle with a 10K. Wendy can cycle 40 miles and you can barely finish 20. So what?

Jealousy and envy are counterproductive and will lead you astray. Run your own race at your own pace, and you'll be setting your own records. When you see others—at the gym, in Spin class, at Pilates—who are stronger, more flexible, thinner or more athletic, be happy for them. Find your serene smile and return your focus to your own situation. Be grateful you have a situation.

You refuse to keep a journal. This may sound like a homework assignment from your dreaded algebra teacher, but the truth is, keeping a journal is a great tool for creating awareness and staying on track. So try it. Just a few observations: what you did; how long you did it; how you felt. Once you have the exercise habit in place, you can stop with the journaling, but if it becomes a habit, it can be a powerful tool for transformation.

You expect quick results. Impatience is a big problem for people just starting to exercise regularly. You expect immediate results, and when you don't see them, you find a reason to quit. Outsmart yourself. Take it day by day. Find joy in just showing up. In time, all the benefits of regular exercise will come your way. It takes the time it takes.

You see yourself as the victim. Many exercise dropouts blame their failure on someone or something else: I can't take time away from my kids. My job is too demanding. I travel too much.

These are excuses created to test your true intention. When you take responsibility for your own health and wellness, you give up being a victim and start living the more active, balanced, joyful life you've always wanted.

The beauty of self-sabotage is that, whatever you do, you can undo. No guilt, no shame, just a willingness to start where you are—this time with a new, improved attitude and greater understanding about what it takes to succeed.

ENERGY EXPRESS-O!   Be a Selfie

"Be yourself; everyone else is already taken."
—Oscar Wilde

GOING DEEPER

Affirmations can sound corny.

"I love and approve of myself."

"I breathe in calmness and breathe out fear."

"I surround myself with people who treat me well."

And yet, they're popular and powerful. You can find hundreds of ready-made affirmations by searching online. Or you can make up your own.

"All is well" always soothes me when I say it, but you may prefer another.

Do affirmations change lives? For some people, the answer is yes.

You won't know until you experiment with a few phrases that feel good to you.

"I can't do this" is a great example of what not to say.

"I'm too tired to go for a walk" is also a no-no. In fact, going for a walk will energize you, so "tired" isn't a feeling you'll have anymore.

Change your thoughts; change your life.

Spinal twists sound like something to avoid. Who wants to twist a knee? An ankle? But spinal twists are different. Done gently, with awareness, they juice up your spine so it stays nourished, supple, spacious. Yoga poses (asanas) were created to bring energy, fluid and freedom to your spine. (Other places, too.) If doctors knew what yogis understand about mindful movement, I'm positive we'd all be healthier, happier, and much more involved with our own healing. We might also have more tattoos.

Twist and Soak.

I try not to talk about yoga with my friend Wendy, because she's started and stopped Hatha yoga so many times. But this time I couldn't resist. I was doing research.

"What do you think's the purpose of all those twisting poses?" I asked.

"I have no idea," she said. "Stretching my laterals?"

Who said ignorance is bliss?

So many smart people just think of yoga as what the poses look like on the outside, focusing on the external form: Triangle, Half-Moon, Down Dog.

Just as important, more important really, is what is going on *inside* your body as you relax into each pose, creating space with your breath, directing energy in ways that restore muscle tone and balance.

Why twist? When you do a twist, you are giving many vital body parts a good squeezing. Followed by a good soaking. This revitalizes your organs, glands, muscles, and joints.

Your kidneys, your adrenals, your liver...different postures work different areas, but the one thing all twists have in common is that they flush out stagnant blood and bring in fresh, healing blood. Twists bring oxygen and vital fluids to your spine, your hips, and your pelvis. Without your help, as the body ages, they shrivel and get stiff and painful from dryness and disuse.

A few twists a day really can help keep the doctor away...from your bank account, for instance.

Learn how. So now you know why you *should* do twists. Next you need to learn *how*. A sensitive, experienced yoga teacher is one good place to begin. You don't want to over-twist, so it's your job to tune in to your body and respect your limits. Every twist isn't safe for everyone. It's one thing to go to your edge; it's another to push through pain. Never do that! And don't let a well-intentioned yoga teacher do it to you.

Now that you're revved up about twisting, why not give it a try?

Susan Winter Ward has written a useful book called "Yoga for the Young at Heart: Accessible Yoga for Every Body." She describes a twist that "lubricates and nourishes the spinal column, increases elasticity of the muscles and ligaments of the spine, balances the nervous system; prevents backache, massages internal organs, toning liver, kidneys and spleen. Aids digestion and elimination."

Amazing! You can't say that about a game of tennis.

What to do. "Sit on the floor, legs out in front of you. Bend your left knee and place your left foot on the floor to the outside of your right thigh. If you feel pain, don't continue. If you continue, ease into the twist slowly, mindfully, feeling your way."

Ward continues: "Inhale deeply as you extend your right arm out to the side, shoulder height.

"Exhaling, bring it around your left knee, holding your knee with the inside of your elbow. Draw the right side of your rib cage toward your inner left thigh.

"Inhale as you raise your left arm up and overhead. Keep your back flat and your heart lifted.

"Exhaling, lower your left hand to the floor behind you, as close to your tailbone as you can. Press the palm of your hand into the floor, lengthening your spine."

More instruction:

"Be sure that both sitting bones stay squarely on the floor.

"Inhale as you lift through the crown of your head and exhale as you rotate your chin to gaze over your left shoulder.

"Press against the floor to lengthen your spine with each inhalation and gently twist a bit more—if possible—with each exhalation, using your front arm and leg as a point of leverage.

"Take three to five long, slow inhalations and exhalations.

"Come out of the pose gently, inhaling as you raise your left arm overhead and exhaling as you bring your body around to face forward again.

"Take a few breaths, and repeat on the other side."

Twists are part of yoga because squeezing and soaking is so good for your body. Once you understand that, you'll find a zillion variations to try—on the floor, in a chair, standing at your desk.

Wherever and whenever you twist, do it with a sense of play and exploration. Some days you'll be tight. Other days you'll feel free. Accept what is, let go of expectations, and be happy you've taken the time to nourish the one and only body you'll ever have.

ENERGY EXPRESS-O! Soak Up the Gratitude

"When you arise in the morning, think of what a privilege it is to be alive—to breathe, to think, to enjoy, to love."
—Marcus Aurelius

GOING DEEPER

Picture your spine.

I mean *really* picture it. The 24 stacked vertebrae (small bones); the soft, gel like cushions called discs that tuck between each vertebrae; the ligaments that connect the bones to the bones; the tendons that connect the muscles to the bones.

Don't collapse; we're just getting started. Each vertebra has a hole in the center so when they all stack up, they form a hollow tunnel that protects the entire spinal cord and its nerve roots.

Imagine those 31 pairs of nerve roots inside the spinal canal, and all the nerve tissue that carries crucial and complex messages from your brain to everywhere else in your body.

But don't stop there. Picture the upper part, the cervical spine, with its seven vertebrae; and the central portion of the spine, the thoracic spine, with its twelve vertebrae; and the lower portion, made up of five or six vertebrae.

Below the lumbar is the sacrum; however, let's return our focus to the spine, and the four basic curves—that's right, four!—and the fact that we depend on our spines to support our body, protect our central nerves, and move us about the planet in remarkable ways.

Our spines make us unique among all animals. Another way we're special is that we can go online and find some animations of the spine in motion, so you can really see what we're talking about. Spineuniverse.com is one place to visit and if you really get hooked on anatomy, check out ADAM.com.

Once you have clarity about your spine, you'll never be bored when you're doing a twist or a stretch. You'll be focused on positioning yourself to bring energizing fluid to every organ, bone, and body part.

Picture that. An open heart, a flexible spine, a strong healthy back for the rest of your life.

I have a highly developed aversion to too much technology. I don't judge others who indulge, and I couldn't live the interesting and blessed life I do without the internet. But the siren call of social media is a concern. "Don't follow me on Facebook," is part of my email signature. I am not on Twitter. I know I shouldn't be shunning social media, especially with a book to promote. I'm being authentic, I tell myself. Moderation in all things. Do I need an intervention?

Tweet Mindfully.

Whenever I see someone texting while driving—Stop that! Pull over!—I start to worry about the cumulative impact of social networking on our brains, our bodies, our fenders, and our nondigital pursuit of a healthy lifestyle.

Tweeting 20 times a day. Texting 50 times a day. Nonstop checking of emails in between. It's a huge time suck, that's for sure. And "not enough time" is the No. 1 excuse people use for eating poorly and not exercising.

But wait! Going online is not the enemy. The internet is a window to the biggest, most fascinating world we've every known. Tweeting has its upside and downside: It discourages empathy and dumbs down deep thinking, but it carries tremendous influence and can work to connect and lift the spirits of people fighting for freedom and justice. Facebook fosters instant, global connections at the same time it redefines and degrades what it is to be—truly, intimately—a friend.

It's complicated. But I'm too young to go back to the quill pen. I have to face up to my confusion and struggle to find the middle way between too much social media and not enough. We all do. And that's why I found Lori Deschene's tweeting advice in Tricycle magazine so helpful.

(Tweeting tips in a major spiritual magazine? Absolutely. Remember, it was the Buddha who said, "If you propose to speak, always ask yourself, is it true, is it necessary, is it kind." But he also knew this: "People with opinions just go around bothering one another.")

Deschene believes in using social media mindfully, as opposed to endlessly. Are you obsessively addicted to email? Do you feel too tied to technology? Are you squeezed for time to live the life you want? Here are some of Deschene's guidelines to help you calm your brain, save your thumbs, and get back in balance:

Practice letting go. It may feel unkind to ignore some tweets or updates, but to be kind to ourselves, we need downtime—time away from technology. Give yourself permission to let yesterday's stream go by.

Be your authentic self. Talk/tweet/email about the things that really matter to you. If you need advice or support, ask for it. Ego-driven tweets focus on an agenda; authenticity communicates from the heart.

Offer random tweets of kindness. Every now and then Deschene asks on Twitter: "Is there anything I can do to help or support you today?" It's her way of connecting personally to followers, her way of giving to others without any expectations in return.

Experience Now, Share Later. Next time you're inclined to snap a picture with your phone, upload it to Facebook, or email it to a friend, pause and reflect: This is keeping me from being in the moment. The less digital narration, the more present you can be.

Be active, not reactive. Instead of having your day constantly interrupted by activity alerts on your social media accounts, decide to choose when and if you want to join the conversation. "Don't expect me to respond to this (email, text, tweet) after 7 p.m. at night" is how one friend of mine handles it.

Enjoy social media. Social media is here to stay. Our job is to use it in a way that helps us feel present and purposeful, not obsessed and addicted. Follow your instincts. If you're a mindful person when you're disconnected from technology, you have all the tools you need to be mindful when you go online.

If these tips sound good to you, but you're not sure how to start, follow the advice of Tim Ferriss, the celebrated author of "The 4-Hour Workweek," a smash hit of a book that has some very good ideas about how to make life less stressful. To cope with the constant crush of email, Ferriss suggests you set up an automatic reply that tells senders you only check your inbox twice a day, at noon and at 4 p.m. Or copy this:

"Thank you for your email. Sadly, it will be deleted. To regain sanity, I am taking a break from email until March. If it is still relevant, please email me again in the month of March."

WHAT! What will people think?

Fear not. If they put down their ever-fidgeting thumbs and *do* think about it, they'll think you're getting your life back under control.

ENERGY EXPRESS-O!   You Talking to Me?

"I am not anti-technology, I am pro-conversation."
—Sherry Turkle

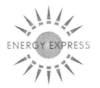

GOING DEEPER

Do you dare notice the amount of time you spend online?

Oh, go ahead. Be brave. Just for fun.

Keep track of how many texts you send in a day, how many times you check your email, how many games you play, videos you watch, social media stuff you post.

It's a cruel thing to ask, I know.

But do it. Just for a day. If possible.

And if it isn't possible, sit back and notice that.

There is a war against breast cancer—and at the same time there is a battle against the war on breast cancer. All that "pink washing" has some people seeing red. Too many nonprofits and businesses are fueling their own growth while the growths that turn into breast cancers continue to affect astonishing numbers of women, and men, too. And now medical authorities tell us that mammograms aren't really useful when it comes to preventing breast cancer and are causing more harm than good. Oops. This is a hot topic for me and every woman I know, which is why it's time to...

Warm Up to Thermograms.

Breast cancer doesn't just run in my family, it gallops. My grandmother, my mother, my sister, my niece, and way too many more women I know and love have all been diagnosed. So when I tell you I keep abreast of this subject, you'll know I'm not just punning you.

And here's what I've discovered about the war on breast cancer that is crucial and has nothing to do with the color pink: Women should take command of their bodies and include thermograms as part of their breast health regimen.

Don't wait for your gynecologist or primary doctor to suggest it. Chances are, they know nothing about this continually improving imaging technology. It's had lousy PR ever since it was approved by the FDA in 1982. Maybe that's because it's simply not part of the billion-dollar cancer industry. Maybe people would care if it had a color of its own...

Breast thermography—using a state-of-the-art digital infrared camera—is safe, effective, involves no radiation or squishing of the breast, and is evolving as a super-important risk-assessment tool for the early detection of breast cancer.

And early detection is everything. "When treated in its earliest stages, most breast cancer has a cure rate of 95 percent," says Dr. Kathryn Ater, a Doctor of Oriental Medicine, who gave me my first, second, and third thermograms over the last several years.

Her mission is simply stated on her Two Birds Thermography website, thermographynewmexico.com: to help women take care of themselves.

"You are the one who decides when and how you're going to monitor your breast health," says Dr. Kate, who's been analyzing thermograms for more than ten years. "Thermography is a tool. It's a piece of the puzzle that we can offer to help find abnormalities in the breast tissue before abnormal growth begins."

Mammograms—and I'm not going to get into all the pros and cons that have women so confused—are simply not useful for early detection.

"A cancer has been growing eight to ten years before it's big enough or dense enough to be detected by mammography," explains Sandra Fields, a Certified Clinical Thermographer with a master's in nursing and 35 years experience in women's health care. She's part of an expanding network of doctors, nurses, patients, and health experts who are spreading the good word about thermograms.

"Women need to know that breast thermography is a promising and safe technology that is a welcome addition to helping women create breast health," says another wise advocate, the best-selling Dr. Christiane Northrup.

The science is simple and makes sense to anyone with a breast or a brain: By the time a tumor is the size of a pinhead (after about two years of growing) it requires its own blood supply. The process of developing that blood supply is called angiogenesis. Thermography is the best technology for detecting angiogenesis because it detects abnormal activity in the breast—increased heat, blood flow, or changing vascular patterns. All of these are early indicators that something suspicious is happening in the breast tissue and needs follow-up.

It's an easy, painless procedure that takes about 30 minutes. The patient stands naked from the waist up, turning in different directions while the technician clicks away, using an infrared thermal camera.

I felt relieved when Dr. Kate went over my most recent thermogram with me. We both looked at the beautiful result, worthy of framing, a swirling psychedelic Peter Max-like pattern of red, blue, green, and yellow.

"Looks good," are the words I remember. She compared the new one with the one from last year. No new vascular supply, no suspicious heat patterns, no new asymmetries.

"Nothing's really changed," she said, and we both knew that's very good news.

I'm not waiting for my insurance company to do the right thing. I pay the $199 out of pocket, and $50 dollars more for Dr. Kate's careful review of the results.

I'm not saying that thermograms can or should replace mammograms. You must decide for yourself. But it is an accurate and reliable first line of defense and prevention, an excellent tool for early detection of a spreading blood supply, and it's not getting the good publicity it merits.

Where is the founder of the Susan G. Komen Foundation when we need her?

ENERGY EXPRESS-O!   Picture This!

"With thermography as your regular screening tool, it's likely that you would have the opportunity to make adjustments to your diet, beliefs, and lifestyle to transform your cells before they become cancerous. Talk about true prevention."
—Christiane Northrup, M.D.

GOING DEEPER

Breast cancer is a subject very near and dear to my heart. Yours, too, probably. Everyone knows someone.

I've made my case. My readers will decide for themselves whether or not to pursue this technology. But whatever you decide, here's something else you can do to help alleviate the breast cancer epidemic and help girls develop into strong, healthy, confident women.

You can engage in what I call fitness philanthropy and support young women who need proven programs and compassionate coaches to help them lead more active, more satisfying lives.

Living a healthier lifestyle is no guarantee that you won't get breast cancer, but there's plenty of evidence to show that girls who grow up eating smart, exercising regularly, learning to cope with stress and deal with fear and anger can lower their risk for developing breast cancer later in life, especially if they get motivated to eat well and avoid obesity.

Girls in the Game works with girls from age 7 to 18, teaching them sports, healthy lifestyle habits, and leadership skills that change their lives in remarkable ways. It's based in Chicago, my hometown, and after 22 years of awards, classroom success, and stunning testimonials from our girls and their families, we're going national, spreading our programs to Baltimore and Dallas. I say "we" because I was the founding chair and I'm still a shameless board member.

So go deeply into GirlsintheGame.org and please support us with time, money, and love.

Told you I was shameless.

One of the saddest developments of the last 40 years is the ginormous rise in childhood obesity. We have sold our children to the junk food vendors and sugary drink manufacturers and—oh, boy and oh, girl—are they paying the price. The number of fat kids more than tripled between 1971 and 2011. Now, about one in three American kids and teens is overweight or obese. All that excess weight puts innocent kids at much greater risk of heart disease, diabetes, cancer, low self-esteem, depression, and early death. It's an epidemic, a national disgrace, and even the best and brightest intentions of former first lady Michelle Obama weren't enough to make Big Food & Big Soda reform their naughty ways. So here's a bit of good news: Some kids are fighting back.

Let Them Eat Rice Cakes.

It can happen in the best of homes. You think you've done everything right as a parent—good schools, restricted screen time, all-cotton underwear—and then one day at dinner, your world explodes.

Your kid goes veggie. She stops eating meat. "I've decided on a plant-based diet," Emma announces out of the blue, turning up her nose, knife, and fork at the beautiful burger on her plate. "How can you eat somebody's mother?"

Some version of this drama plays out every day in homes across America, as more young people become aware of the face on the plate, and how it relates to the planet they live on.

Kids eating green is trending up, and meatloaf-loving parents need help, strategies, patience, sometimes pharmaceuticals.

Step one? Don't panic. There are experts to advise you and one of them is Lisa Barley, writing in Vegetarian Times, a great resource for 100 things to do with chickpeas.

"Your child's new diet doesn't have to make your life more difficult," she explains in language meant to calm you. There are ways to be supportive, less stressed. Here are some of them, along with my own embellishments:

Don't worry. Your kids health won't suffer if they're following a well-planned veggie diet, say the authorities, including the American Academy of Pediatrics. They can get all the vitamins and minerals they need to be healthy and strong, but it requires some study and effort.

Listen up. Ask your kids to share the reasons they're giving up meat, Lisa suggests. Keep an open mind. If they've gone on YouTube and seen the horrible things that happen to cows and chicken in the name of factory farming, take a look yourself. Sit down over a plate of edamame and talk it over. More important than talking is *listening* to your child. Listening without judging.

"Think of it as an opportunity to get to know their values and worldview," Lisa Barley writes.

Assign homework. Lisa wants you to get your kids involved in whatever eating changes they want to make. Have your newbie vegetarian "make a list of nutritious snacks and meals, and draft a shopping list, " she says in a state of mind some parents will regard as delusional.

Another strategy: Go over the vegetarian food pyramid together, so all involved can see what a well-balanced diet looks like. In case your vegetarian food pyramid has gone missing, you can always find it again at vegetariannutrtion.org/food pyramid.pdf.

Be a student. When a child goes veggie, it's smart to have a couple of reliable resources you can turn to with your questions and concerns. But beware! There is a lot of confusing, conflicting and corporately designed nutrition information online. Lisa recommends parents check in with two nonprofits I've trusted and admired for years: Oldways Vegetarian Network and Physicians Committee for Responsible Medicine.

Set ground rules. Rule No. 1: "Make it clear that junk food vegetarianism won't fly," Lisa says. Eating real food should be the focus, not bags of chips and cookies that are marked vegan and packed with sugar. If you need help with meal planning and prep, ask your child to pitch in. (Why do I hear you laughing?)

And keep the drama over food choices to a minimum. Declare the dining table a no-war zone. Nothing puts a bigger chill in the air than a heated discussion about tortured and stressed industrial chickens...while half the family is chewing on them.

Cook and eat together. I've saved the best for last. It's also the most idealistic, but so what? Help create a world where everyone respects everyone else's food choices. Start in your own kitchen. Focus on foods you can all eat together, like make-your-own tacos with different fillings. Or pasta with one meat sauce, one veggie sauce. DIY pizza is good, too.

The crucial thing is your attitude. A kid choosing to go meatless isn't the end of the world. It's an introduction to a world you might want to join yourself someday.

As one mother told Lisa, "There are many bad choices that a child can make in this world, and being a vegetarian is definitely not one of them."

ENERGY EXPRESS-O!   LOL

"Vegetarian—that's an old Indian word meaning
lousy hunter."
—Andy Rooney

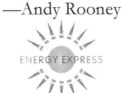

GOING DEEPER

Getting your young ones kids to make healthy food choices is right up there with climbing Mt. Everest, in high heels and a burkini.

It's challenging. But it's not impossible. One strategy is to cozy up to your kid and read aloud from Michael Pollan's classic "Food Rules," a small book that can have a huge impact on your entire family's eating habits and poundage.

—"If it came from a plant, eat it; if it was made in a plant, don't."

—"It's not food if it arrived through the window of your car."

—"The whiter the bread, the sooner you'll be dead."

—"Eat animals that have themselves eaten well."

And what third-grader won't love this one?

—"Avoid food products containing ingredients that a third-grader can't pronounce."

Pollan's book works well for kids because he's written it in a simple and straightforward style, stripping away all the hard science, the biochemistry, the thermodynamically complex descriptions of insulin and fat metabolism.

Instead he artfully delivers 64 rules that are fun to read and easy to digest. Here's a sampling, just to whet your appetite for the real thing:

"Eat (real) food." Every year, about 17,000 new products show up on grocery shelves, and most of them are so anti-health they shouldn't even be called food. Pollan calls them "edible food-like substances" and "industrial novelties." Avoid them, and watch how much better you feel.

"Avoid food products containing ingredients that no ordinary human would keep in the pantry." When was the last time you ran to the store for another box of ammonium sulfate? Or ethoxylated diglycerides? These additives are there to prolong shelf life, not your life. Stay away.

"Avoid foods that are pretending to be something they are not." Imitation butter, imitation (nonfat) cream cheese, soy-based mock meats...

Just say no.

And this final one:

"Don't eat breakfast cereals that change the color of your milk." Why? Because those are the cereals that are highly processed and full of refined carbohydrates and chemical additives.

What 10-year-old can resist seeing what happens with his next bowl of Coco Pops?

People die. Loved ones are miserable. How do you comfort the grieving? It's something to think about, learn about, offer up to your brokenhearted friends. One thing I know to be true in my 40 years tracking healthy lifestyle habits is that the more you learn about death, the greater your pleasure in life. Then, you're not afraid to engage with the inevitable. You actually want to. Loving life isn't a state of denial and death isn't the enemy; it's the star you navigate by to lead the life you'll leave, fully and authentically.

Bring Life to Death.

Dealing with death—your own, a loved one's, the death of a child—is a required course at the University of Wellness, Ballet, and Refrigeration.

No one gets out of here alive. This we know. What we don't know is everything else. Death is the biggest mystery of all, leaving many of us clueless when it comes to comforting someone who's lost a loved one.

What do you say? What *don't* you say? Do you mention the dead person by name? Do you try to offer good advice, to be helpful and loving?

"Do *not* give advice," advises Edie Hartshorne, a master of social work, longtime therapist, former Fulbright Scholar and award-winning author of "Light in Blue Shadows," a wise and inspiring book about death, compassion, and transforming grief.

After her 20-year-old son, Jonathan, died unexpectedly, Edie went on a dark and deep journey into her own pain and unraveling. When she came out the other side and wrote her book—"a journey of loss and grief that leads to a place of wonder," says Isabel Allende on the jacket cover—Edie had a new awareness of many things, including what it means to comfort, and be comforted.

"Many times when we feel uncomfortable with another person's loss, we offer advice, hoping to make everything better."

Resist, says Edie. The person grieving doesn't need advice. She needs to be heard, to have her loss acknowledged. She needs her friends, her family, to be fully present, listening to whatever she has to say.

Here are some more empowering Edie-isms to help you through the inevitable:

Don't say you know just how the grieving person feels. You don't! So don't equate or compare your grief to the other person's. When you say, "I know just how it is. I lost my mom a year ago," it can trivialize the other person's pain.

"This can be particularly true when a parent has lost a child," Edie writes. "It's better to make no comparisons."

Don't remain silent. Very often, because we fear saying the wrong thing, we say nothing at all about the truth of what's going on. That's a mistake, Edie counsels. It's isolating for the person who's grieving to be surrounded by silent friends.

"It's so important to validate the other person's reality," she writes. Share your truth plainly. "I just heard your terrible news. I am so sorry and sad. I just want you to know I am holding you in my heart." Say it your way, with your true voice, but don't hide in silence.

Don't try to fix your friend or family member. This goes along with "not giving advice," but you can't hear it often enough: "There is nothing to fix," Edie writes. It's natural for someone to feel grief when a loved one dies, and it's very painful.

Your work is to "stay present to the other person's pain." Just be there. It's not your job to solve anything.

Don't ask, "Is there anything I can do?" Just do it. Take the initiative. When people grieve, Edie says, they're often too overwhelmed to sort out what needs to be done, or too shy to ask for help.

Notice what needs to be done and take action: Bring over dinner; drop off flowers; walk the dog. This requires a sensitive touch, but if you wait to be asked, you may miss the opportunity to truly help.

Rather than focusing on the don'ts, embrace what you can do for your loved ones in times of grief. These do's are closer to Edie Hartshorne's true nature. She's a poet, a musician, and a very positive person:

Be present to exactly where your grieving friend is in the moment. If six months have passed, and he suddenly bursts into tears, "take a deep breath to bring yourself fully into the moment," says Edie. "Listening fully and with a big heart is the most powerful medicine."

Make phone calls to your friend or family members during that first year. Grieving people are achingly aware of the birthdays and anniversaries involving the person who died. Say something! It feels very lonely when those dates go by unacknowledged.

ENERGY EXPRESS-O!   Everything Changes

"Life and death are of extreme importance. Time swiftly passes by and opportunity is lost. Each of us should strive to awaken. Awaken! Take heed, do not squander your life."
—Eihei Dogen

GOING DEEPER

Do what Edie suggests—call a friend who's lost a loved one this past year.

It may be difficult for you, but don't be afraid to do it.

Make the call with the intention of listening, not talking.

Listen without interrupting. Allow for silent moments, without feeling discomfort. Let the conversation unfold. You're not calling to fix anything.

When you hang up, you'll feel very good that you made the call.

And so will your friend.

And that's what compassion looks like.

Autumn

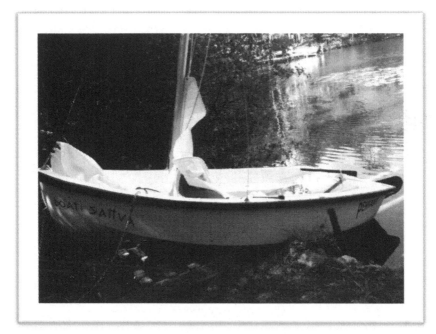

North Woods, Wisconsin

"Delicious Autumn!
My very soul is wedded to it, and if I were a bird
I would fly about the earth seeking
consecutive autumns."
—George Eliot

"Autumn calls us to a still and silent place and
beckons us to sit back and observe a little deeper."
—Natalie Goldberg

"There is something so special in the early leaves
drifting from the trees —as if we are all allowed a
chance to peel, to refresh, to start again."
—Ruth Ahmed

How do you maintain a healthy weight? It's so personal, so painful for so many. Not my mother. She was zaftig and beautiful, and she never tortured herself with diets. "Never go on a diet," she told me while I was still young enough to have her chocolate cake and milk for breakfast every day. "You'll only gain it all back and more." All the research on dieting has proven her right. I was a junior size 15-16 when I graduated from high school and now I'm not. And that's because eventually I learned how truly wise my mother was. The chocolate cake for breakfast thing? No one's perfect.

Know Your Body Chemistry.

It's sad to see so many people in the country crippled and confused by the food they eat. It's the fake foods that make us fat, and the real foods that our bodies thrive on. Yet Big Food thrives on selling us cheap, manufactured fare, so obesity overtakes us, and we're left with crumbs.

What to do? Go see a nutritionist. This is what I find myself telling countless people—family, friends, total strangers on airplanes—in spite of all I know about the fruitlessness of giving advice. Add a nutritionist to your health team. A gifted body worker is good, too, but a savvy nutritionist is worth her weight in avocados.

Here's why it's so crucial: Your body chemistry—the building blocks of your health and well-being—is uniquely your own. Yes! Just like your fingerprints, only different, because your fingerprints stay the same, but your nutritional profile is something you can transform in weeks…if you really want to.

But you have to proceed with caution. We are constantly being seduced by what we see on TV, in magazines, online 24/7. Need strength? Energy? Take this multivitamin! Chew this calcium! Swallow this glowing green drink!

Maybe you need it, maybe you don't. Not even Dr. Oz can tell you what nutrients to add or subtract until you discover what your own levels are right now. High in cholesterol? Low in vitamin B-12? Simple blood and urine tests will tell the tale. Eureka! Then what?

Many health experts don't know beans about nutrition. And yet, if you don't feed your body what it needs—the proper mix of nutrients, from antioxidants to zinc—it will, over time, underperform, get sick, and fall apart. It's that simple.

But figuring out how to get the nutrients we need to digest our food, support our hearts, nourish our brains, resist disease and inflammation, and promote good health and energy has become incredibly confusing.

If sugar is so lethal in excess—and it is—why is it packed into so many of our processed foods? Why is olive oil good and fake butter blends bad? Why is it so important to limit low-net carbs and get your body to burn fat instead of glucose?

That's why a consultation and continuing relationship with a nutritionist is such a satisfying experience. The good ones know which foods help us heal and which make us sick. They can help us help ourselves cut back on sugar and understand the importance of healthy fats. Together, you can fine-tune your body chemistry, using real food and drink instead of exotic fasts, cleanses, and unnecessary supplements.

They also can tell you if you have any imbalances—too acidic or too alkaline, too much iron or too little—and customize an eating plan that moves you toward better memory, a mightier metabolism, and fewer burps and belches.

So why isn't this kind of vital-to-the-core nutritional counseling commonly covered by our medical insurance? It's crazy! It's also an indication of how sick our drug-centered health care system is. The Affordable Care Act looks more kindly on wellness and prevention, but, as of printing, is in the process of being overturned. What comes next? No one knows. But if nutritional counseling is part of the new system, I'll be shocked.

Whatever...this is your wake-up call. You really *are* what you eat. Sit down with an experienced, enlightened nutritionist and review your body chemistry, one on one, vitamin by mineral, protein by fat, so you are less likely to suffer from obesity, diabetes, cancer and other forms of nutritional neglect.

Do not, I warn you, try this with your family doctor. I know that's changing a bit, but still, the vast majority of our docs still treat illness with drugs, not lifestyle change. It's hard to blame them, because that *is* what's taught in medical school. It's what drug companies prefer, too, but don't get me started on that or I'll never get back to the subject, which is this: If you're really ready to change your life, then partner up with a nutritionist.

That said, I must now confess: until a few years ago, I'd never been to one myself. I've interviewed them, gone to workshops, read their books, praised the role they play in wellness and weight control, but I'd never actually consulted with one—my body chemistry, her big brain—before.

And then I met professor Carmen Fusco, clinical nutritionist and research scientist, who has a remarkable understanding of the healing power of food. I nearly cried after my first two-hour session with her, and not just because I had to pay out-of-pocket. She's a genius!

And now I want everyone I know to find his or her own Carmen Fusco, assuming we can't clone her, which she wouldn't like at all.

ENERGY EXPRESS-O!   This Is No Yolk

"Marilynn! Look at your white cell count. You're fighting a virus! I want you adding turmeric to your eggs!"
—Carmen Fusco

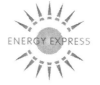

GOING DEEPER

I know what you're wondering: How do I find a really good nutritionist?

It could be a challenge, but you're up to it. You just need an appetite for change.

Don't be discouraged if your doctor can't facilitate your search. The nurse at the front desk is likely to be a better bet.

Put out your own feelers. Talk to informed friends; search the internet; check in with local holistic health centers; join an integrative medical practice that makes an honored place for nutritional guides and wellness coaches.

If I were suddenly dropped into a strange city with no friends and a dead mobile phone, and I was networking for a reliable nutritionist, I'd go over to the best yoga center in town and study the community bulletin board.

They're out there.

Once you and your nutritionist figure out the biochemistry of what your body needs—and you are finally ready to do the work of making change happen—the endless spiral of dieting, deprivation, and depression can come to an end.

After 40 years on the fitness beat, I've developed a healthy skepticism about medical care in the United States. It serves too few and costs too much. Preventable medical errors are the third leading cause of death in America—death from medical care itself! Our mainstream M.D.'s are a mixed bag. Some can save your life. Others can kill you. Overmedicating is standard. To be wary is to be wise. I learned that and a whole lot more reading a fascinating book by the fearless and famous Dr. Jerome Groopman.

Team Up With Your Doctor.

Who likes going to the doctor? Exactly no one...especially if you have something we all dread—symptoms!

A sudden chest pain, a nagging backache, a persistent headache. Though the symptoms will vary, your goal is always the same. You want your physician to figure our what's wrong. And you want to get well. Fast.

And that's why Dr. Jerome Groopman's award-winning classic, "How Doctors Think," is so valuable. He teaches us to be a better patient. He recognizes that doctors are far from perfect. They make mistakes, and the majority of errors they make are not technical screwups, but rather errors in thinking.

Doctors are under great pressure to perform, and perform quickly, Groopman explains. They jump to conclusions they're comfortable with. They ignore facts that don't fit. They have egos and emotions that can cloud their judgment and lead them astray. In short, they're just like us.

So how can you avoid those problems and hugely improve the quality of your medical care? Here are some highlights from "How Doctor's Think":

Be a partner. You can't be passive or shy or intimidated by your doctor. To lower your risk of a wrong diagnosis, Groopman says, you must be engaged and involved.

"Patients and their loved ones can be true partners with physicians when they know how their doctors think and why doctors sometimes fail to think."

Trust your instincts. If you sense your doctor is rushing through your exam, or isn't listening to your story, or just plain doesn't like you, pay attention.

"Research shows that patients do pick up on a doctor's negativity, but few understand how that affects their care, and they rarely change doctors." Groopman's advice? Change doctors!

Don't be pigeonholed. Doctors think in stereotypes: the hysterical housewife, the overworked executive, the kooky hypochondriac. If you think your doctor isn't paying enough attention to who you really are and what you're saying, call him or her on it.

Be informed. It's OK, even desirable, to learn everything you can about your case "and respectfully question each and every assumption about the diagnosis and treatment."

You do this not because you don't trust the doctor, or hospital, Groopman writes, "but because God did not make people omniscient."

Ask questions. "What we say to a physician and how we say it sculpts his thinking. That includes not only our answers, but our questions."

You can positively influence your doctor's thinking by asking smart questions: "What else could it be?" "Is there anything that doesn't fit?" "Is it possible I have more than one problem?"

If your doctor doesn't have time for your questions, and isn't capable of giving clear answers, find a better doctor.

Slow down the process. Studies have shown that physicians, on average, give their patients only 18 seconds to tell their story before they interrupt. Yikes. You spend more time ordering a venti, extra-hot, sugar-free, five shots, no foam, pumpkin-spice latte at Starbucks.

If your doctor is distracted—interrupted by staff, looking at the clock or a computer—speak up.

"The inescapable truth is that good thinking takes time. Working in haste and cutting corners are the quickest routes to cognitive errors."

Beware of corrupt practices. It's well-known but still shocking: Some doctors get financial incentives or kickbacks to prescribe certain drugs or do suspect surgeries. "Spinal fusion may be the radical mastectomy of our time," Groopman writes.

Ask hard questions, and pursue second opinions. And please distrust any doctor who tries to turn the natural aging process into a disorder.

Every year, more than 250,000 Americans die from medical errors. You don't want to be one of them. It's a life-saving cliche: The best defense is a good offense. Find a doctor you trust and respect and can partner with. Be involved. Ask questions. Take a friend with you to take notes and listen.

And, finally, don't be intimidated by the white coat and framed medical degrees. Your doctor went to medical school. You didn't. But you've been thinking things though your whole life. Don't stop now. Start where you are. Learn what you need to know. And if she calls you by your first name, you do the same.

ENERGY EXPRESS-O!   The Art of Medicine

"My doctor is wonderful. Once when I couldn't afford an operation, he touched up the X-rays."
—Joey Bishop

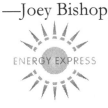

GOING DEEPER

If your doctor isn't willing to partner with you in the way Dr. Groopman describes, find one who is.

They're out there. Do the research. Ask around, and look for key words to clue you in to a practice that combines the best of Western and Eastern practices: integrative medicine, complementary medicine, patient-centered medicine.

You want docs, nurses, physician assistants, therapists, nutritionists, and assorted practitioners who trained to take into account your whole being, a team who invite and encourage your involvement. You need them to be good listeners, not just prescription-writing machines. You can expect them to take the time it takes to make a proper diagnosis, and then stay involved, with impeccable follow through.

And find a doctor who doesn't see death as a failure, a doctor who isn't afraid to talk to you knowledgeably and compassionately about end-of-life issues.

Remember: The medical system in the U.S. is a for-profit system. It can be life-saving, it can be genius, but it is focused on treating illness, not preventing it. Your well-being depends on both, so don't settle for less.

I'm a real foodie when it comes to real food, and dining out in evolved, delicious, and conversation-friendly restaurants is one of the pleasures of my life. It's also a minefield. Portions are crushing. And food sources are suspect. How do I know my wild trout wasn't raised in a swimming pool? Join me in the sport of Menu Aerobics, an exercise in awareness for people with an appetite for knowing more, and eating a little less.

Mind Your Menus.

Dining out has become our national pastime. So has porking up. Is there a link between the two? You bet your burgers. We're a fast-food nation of overeating eater-outers, and if you want to trim down and stay healthy, you might want to line up for personal instruction in one of my favorite sports: Menu Aerobics.

It's played sitting down, using your hands, with an assist from your nimble brain. The playing field is every restaurant on Earth. The only skill you need is mindfulness. Eating out isn't the enemy. Spacing out is.

Split meals. When did portions in American restaurants explode? It's obscene. Europeans gasp at our super-size meals. Asians faint. We're one of the fattest nations in the world, with the heart disease and diabetes to prove it. And research supports the obvious: The more food on your plate, the more you eat.

So share an entree with someone else, preferably at your own table. Even if there's an annoying split plate charge, it's worth it. More and more, smart restaurants are offering up half orders or smaller portions. Train yourself to order less. Tell yourself you can always order more if you're still hungry. (You won't be.)

Focus on starters. Advanced players skip over the entrees. Instead, they focus on the appetizers, sides and salads. That's where the gold is. The food's still a taste thrill, the portions are more manageable, and, yes, the prices are lower.

You'll also save hundreds of calories when you make a meal from two appetizers or one starter and a salad, but calorie counting isn't the point. It's not as irritating as texting at the table, but it can ruin the pleasure of the meal. When you eat, eat. Slow down. Chew. Savor every bite. Guilt around food is counterproductive, and it actually promotes indigestion.

Waist not, want not. Menu Aerobics is played best with a doggy bag. You order the entree you want, eat half, and take the rest home. If you meet a hungry person or stray animal on the way, bingo! If you resist taking leftovers because they tend to turn to pond scum at the back of the fridge, accept yourself as you are, and if no one else wants your half-portion of chicken tikka vindaloo, leave it on the table—with a nice tip for your server, just to help close the gap.

Skip over fried. Menu Aerobics gives you the core strength to glide quickly past the deep fried stuff: the fried chicken, the fried fish, alas, the fried cheese balls.

It's not a matter of "bad" food as much as a bad habit. (Tasty, though.) When you have a lapse—and you will—and you wind up with a plate of fried onion rings the size of a Chihuahua, at least pull off some of the breading.

This is extremely challenging in the case of crispy french fries, my weakness and my strength. I know I love them; I refuse to give them up. So I ask for the salt, count out nine beauties, (not out loud), and hope to be conscious of every bite.

Then I move the rest out of reach.

(Full disclosure: I've been known to reach over three dinner plates to grab another handful of crispy fries but please, do as I say, not as I do, unless you're willing to take responsibility for your actions. I am when it comes to fries, especially if I can get them with spicy Dijon mustard.)

Say the mantra. Memorize this phrase until it rolls off your tongue without the slightest embarrassment:

"Dressing on the side, please."

Was that so hard?

Practice at home, and repeat it with a smile in every restaurant you visit. I'm all for tasty sauces and dressings, but many places pour on way too much and without thinking, you soak it all in.

Instead, dip your fork in, and sprinkle lightly.

Do you need bread? Some Menu Aerobic practitioners shun the buns and ask waiters to take the breadbasket away. Too many calories, too much gluten, too bloating. If you can't resist, satisfy yourself with a few bites or crusts. If you want butter—and who doesn't?—make a little go a long way.

Ordering wine? If you're not interested, fine, but if you are, savor every sip of the best wine you can afford and exercise moderation. Then you can toast your good judgment, repeatedly, throughout the night.

Dessert! Talk about a minefield. Menu Aerobics doesn't require you to deny, deprive, punish. You already know that the healthiest dessert is fresh fruit, but there are genius pastry chefs out there determined to defeat your game plan. So, order one gorgeous caramel coated brownie with two scoops of pecan green tea ice cream, and pass it around the table. Take the first bite, or the last bite, and kiss it goodbye.

ENERGY EXPRESS-O! Hold the Syrup

"I went to a restaurant that serves 'breakfast at any time.' So I ordered French toast during the Renaissance."
—Steven Wright

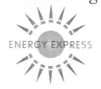

GOING DEEPER

This is a biggie. It's the opposite of eating out.

Here it is: Learn to cook, and eat at home more often.

How will you make this happen? Trial and error? Online videos? Meal Kits from NYT Cooking? The Food Channel?

Cooking tasty meals, at home, using real ingredients and simple recipes, is not difficult. It doesn't have to be time-consuming either. If there's a will, there's a way...so let me weigh in with this easy-as-pie idea.

This week, find a recipe for an entree that makes your heart sing, your mouth water. Carmelized onions under giant white beans with spinach and feta. Wild salmon with figs. Scrambled eggs with mushrooms and goat cheese. Add a veggie or two. Maybe a big salad. Invite some friends over to cook with you,

What you prepare isn't as important as the act of doing it, together.

And if you can get your kids to join you in food prep, on a regular basis, you'll earn frequent cooker miles and a permanent place in the Parenting Hall of Fame.

I keep a little pink Post-it note on my laptop, just to the left of the track pad. When it gets wrinkled and worn, I make a new one. It says, "Do The Practice." It's a reminder, an old-school version of the Apple watch that taps your wrist when it's time to stand up. Standing up is part of my practice. So is sitting still, doing yoga, race walking, somatics, red wine, and sweet conversation at sunset. What's your practice? If you don't have one yet, don't worry. But when you do, make a little note for yourself and leave it where you can see it everyday. It doesn't have to be pink.

Do the Practice.

Looking to boost your well-being? I'm a big believer in home gyms. If you can't play out in nature, then hitting your home gym is the next best thing. You wake up, throw on what passes for workout clothes, and before you can find an excuse to skip it, you're walking the treadmill or riding the stationary bike or pumping the weights and spreading joy throughout your body.

Yes! What could be better? No time-sucking commute to the gym. No monthly dues. No comparing your self to the thinner and more buffed all around you. (Never, ever do that.)

At home, it's just you and the practice and your growing awareness that regular exercise is the rock-solid foundation of a healthy lifestyle. You'll gain strength, reduce stress, and you'll keep your joints juiced in a way that helps with agility and balance.

Exercising at home burns pounds of calories. But keep in mind: You can't outrun your fork. If weight loss is your goal, a home gym is a dear friend, but it's no substitute for smaller portions and a ban on processed foods and sugary cola drinks, especially the ones with fake sweeteners.

So make space, even if it's the corner of your bedroom or a portion of the family room, and, need I mention, far from the fridge.

Make it inviting. Your work out space can be small, but if it's nasty—a dirty basement, a stuffy attic, a chilly garage—you'll find a reason to avoid it.

An area with natural light, fresh air and no clutter is the feng shui ideal, but if that's not possible, start where you are. Make your space clean and appealing. A yoga mat and a fresh flower in your living room can work wonders on your mind and body. Whatever the size, treat it like the sacred space it is.

Feel good about what you spend. I don't know your budget for home gear, but two things I do know for sure: First, investing in your own wellness is money well-spent. And second, don't buy cheap stuff. It will feel junky, and you won't use it. If you've got $5,000 or more to outfit an entire room, be thankful, but you can get just as fit for $500 or less, using free weights, stability balls, jump ropes, resistance bands, etc. It's easier than ever to find high-quality used gear—online, in specialty stores—but it's best to try it before you buy it, to make sure everything feels good and sturdy.

Plan for cardio, stretching, strengthening. For a balanced workout, your home gym should have at least one solid piece of aerobic equipment (a bike, a treadmill, an elliptical cross-trainer, your choice), plus space and gear for stretching and strengthening. If you're new to exercising, buy some time with a personal trainer (or consult with books,

DVDs, etc.) and get started on a home routine that will safely deliver the results you want.

Make it user-friendly. Equip your space with whatever it takes to make your workout enjoyable. Music can be a great motivator. Exercise purists believe that watching TV or reading a book is a distraction. To get into the zone of peak performance, they advise you concentrate your attention on your inner body, your breathing. I know that's sound advice, but I also know how much I enjoy pedaling my recumbent bike while going through my magazine pile or talking back to the news shows. Better to ride to Rachel Maddow than never pedal at all.

Retreating to a workout space you've created mindfully—embellishing it with photos you love, stones you've kept, quotes that inspire you—will exert a powerful influence on your willingness to come back to it.

And don't forget to add a meditation pillow to the mix, even if you're not sure what to do with it. Someday, if you keep your brain healthy and curious, you'll sit down on it.

Keep a journal. To make the most of your home gym, show up every day. Keep a notebook, even if it's just a few lines. Jot down the date, what you did and how you felt. If writing intimidates you, do it anyway.

Why? Keeping track in a journal is an ancient and highly effective magic trick when it comes to making change. It focuses you. It creates awareness. It will help you develop the habit of a regular exercise practice. I promise you that when that happens, your whole life will change in remarkable and delicious ways.

ENERGY EXPRESS-O!   The Tao of Pooh

"A bear, however hard he tries, grows tubby
without exercise."
—A.A. Milne

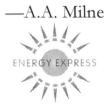

GOING DEEPER

Here's a question I hear a lot: When is the best time to do a home practice?

Is it early in the morning, when you're fresh and perky and want to wake up your body and mind to the whole day ahead of you?

Or is it later in the day, after work, after you've made a thousand little decisions and your body is desperate to unload some of the stress?

Here's the answer: The best time to do a home practice is a personal choice. When do you feel like doing it? When can you make time? When does it feel more like pleasure than punishment?

It may vary from day to day. That's OK, too. Some people use exercise to tire themselves out at night, to help them sleep. Others wouldn't dare jump on the treadmill after dinner because it gets the mojo going in a way that makes it harder to put it to bed.

There is no one best time to exercise. There is only the time that works best for you, this day, this moment. If it varies, let it vary. Just do the practice.

And if you miss a day, no sweat. Come back to it the next day. Begin. Again.

As your birthdays come and go, so might your interest in extreme rock climbing. It's OK to adjust our sports as we age. In fact, it's preferable if you want to have what yogis call "a sustainable practice." So I'm introducing the idea of returning to a sport you once loved, now a better learner, now a slower go-er. The goal is to be a life-long learner, adjusting when you have to so you can stay active, curious, and useful for as long as you can. When that's no longer possible? We want grace. As my friend Ana likes to say, "Walking, talking, dead."

Rediscover an Old Love.

I fell in love with the joy and thrills of cross-country skiing all over again on a recent back country holiday in the spectacular mountains of Pagosa Springs, Colorado. I swear it had nothing to do with the local cannabis dispensary.

The snow conditions were perfect, my companions were high-spirited, and I had the joy of re-learning a sport that is considered one of the greatest workouts there is.

I used to cross-country ski in the North Woods of Wisconsin, but then I moved to the Western mountains and downhill skiing swept me off my feet. Repeatedly. Eventually, I gained new skills and became a solid intermediate skier with no interest whatsoever in going steeper, faster, bumpier.

"I like slow skiing," I used to tell my instructors, who never believed me. "I don't care about speed. I care about fun."

Learning to ski downhill gave me strength, confidence, balance, and edge control. It also gave me a concussion last year on an easy blue run—I slid headfirst

into a rock, crushed my helmet, escaped a crippling injury—
and decided in the emergency room to give cross-country
skiing another go.

It was fabulous! No lines, no snowboarders, no $100
lift tickets. And no need for helmets. I'm not ready to ditch
downhill, but I am inspired to tell you five things about
cross-country skiing to encourage you to try it yourself:

An amazing workout. Downhill skiing won't
develop your cardiovascular fitness; cross-country skiing will.
You'll strengthen your heart and lungs, not to mention your
legs, arms, shoulders, back and core. Cross-country is a
highly efficient aerobic sport, rhythmical and repetitive,
requiring continuous effort, building endurance as you go.
Downhill is a controlled fall down a mountain. In fact, if you
want to downhill safely and well, you'll get in shape *before* you
hit the slopes. And as a calorie-burner, cross-country beats
downhill every step of the way. Every limb, every joint, is in
motion, and you get the bonus of working your body in a
cross-over fashion—right leg forward, left arm forward; left
leg forward, right arm forward—that works both sides of
your brain in a coordinated, balanced, blissful way.

Consider the cost. Cross-country skiing costs much
less than downhill, so you can afford to do it more often.
The best cross-country boots cost a third of what downhill
boots cost, and they are 1,000 times more comfortable. A
day pass to use groomed trails might cost 10 bucks
compared to $40-to-$100 dollars or more to go downhill.
And lessons! Learning to downhill ski can take years. You
can absorb the basics of cross-country in a lesson or two,
and then practice, practice, practice. And then there's the
cost of hurting yourself. Downhill skiing is considered a
high-risk, high injury sport. Cross-country isn't. The pace is
slower, but the pay off can be just as thrilling.

Fun for the whole family. I've heard it said that if you can walk, you can cross-country ski. It's not exactly true because there are skills involved, and you need to learn them to maximize your fun and minimize your risk. But just about anyone can earn to cross-country ski, so the 8-year-olds and 80-year-olds can play together, instead of just meeting for lunch.

The gear has improved. Backcountry cross-country skiing—ungroomed trails on wider skis, with edges—is giving new life to cross-country, and so is skate skiing. My new backcountry skis are much lighter (and shorter) than my old ones. It makes the uphills much easier and the downhills more controllable. Learning to snow plow is essential no matter what your gear, and the newer, lighter skis with edges make that much easier, too.

You connect to nature. When you downhill ski, you need to focus full attention on your technique, your turns, and avoiding trouble. The margin for error is small. When you cross-country ski, not so much. It's slower, less risky, more meditative. You can look around, absorb the beauty, appreciate nature in all her winter splendor. Part of the magic of cross-country is the regular, repetitive breathing—slow, steady, deep. It takes you to another place, physically, mentally, spiritually.

I can't wait to go back.

ENERGY EXPRESS-O!   Keep Smiling

"Cross-country skiing is great if you live in a small country."
—Steven Wright

ENERGY EXPRESS

GOING DEEPER

If you can walk, you can cross-country ski. That's what I was told the first time I ventured out, and I believed it. Wrong. Cross-country skiing—one of the great workouts of the world—is a challenging aerobic sport. Don't expect it to come to you naturally, the way walking does.

So sign up for a few cross-country lessons, rent the equipment, give it a try.

But resist giving it just *one* try.

If your body isn't used to the stride, the glide, the engaged core, the balance, it may rebel at first, screaming: "This is too hard. I can't do this. I want to stop!"

If and when that happens, shift away from the negative and slow down. Way down. Look around and notice how white the snow is, the brilliance of the sky, the sound your skis make when you press down on your forward leg.

Go back to your breath, listening to the sound of the inhale, the release of the exhale.

Find pleasure in the rhythm, the flow: forward and backward, side to side, moment to moment.

You may find that cross-country skiing isn't your sport.

But then again, you may strike gold.

The U.S. government is doing a pathetic job of keeping us safe from harmful foods and pesticides, toxic cosmetics and chemicals, polluted air, and yucky water. Capitalism invests in bottom-line profits, and there's a fortune to be made in processed food, unnecessary personal care products, and nonstick cookware that makes cleanup easier and health problems more likely. It's a deep, dark, overgrown jungle out there in Consumer Protection Land. And Roundup is not the answer. So, dear reader, until there is an answer...

Be Your Own Uncle Sam.

On the Healthy Lifestyle beat, you can't ignore politics. Well, you can, but it would be wrong.

Think about it: Personal health is hugely influenced by public policy. The air we breathe, the water we drink, the poisons in our plastics, the toxins in our toiletries are all health threats to be reckoned with. The government does its best, whatever that means, but the best is not good enough when it comes to your well-being. Vigilance is called for—now more than ever.

And, still, there is hope. During President Obama's final year in office, Congress was finally having a go at redoing the shoddy and shameful Toxic Substances Control Act. It was passed in 1976 to the delight of the chemical industry, and should have been called the Toxic Substances Out of Control Act.

Our tainted environment—from lakes to lipsticks, from off-gassing furniture to off-gassing cows—is widely considered a public health calamity. It's so bad that Republicans and Democrats were reaching across the aisle in

2016, not just to strangle each other, but to stop the incoming missile that is the marketing of dangerous products to consumers.

The decades of research leading to possible Congressional reform is above reproach and downright frightening. Synthetic (manmade) chemicals in our cosmetics, food, furniture, household cleaners, plastic bottles, toys, water—pretty much everything—are irrefutably linked to a hideously wide variety of cancers, heart disease, obesity, male infertility, ADHD, and—that should be enough to catch your attention.

"Of the more than 80,000 chemicals currently used in the United States," says the National Resources Defense Council, "most have not been adequately tested for their effect on human health."

And how about this read-it-slowly summary by the Environmental Defense Fund: "One of three formulated products sold by major retailers contains chemicals known to pose health risks."

Yikes. The EPA hasn't been testing, and the chemical industry hasn't been resting, and it's all gotten so dangerous, so threatening to our health and safety, even Congress paid attention.

The Lautenberg Chemical Safety Act shifts the burden of proof onto the chemical companies, so they have to honestly prove a chemical is safe before it can be sold to and used by humans. They don't have to do that now. Isn't that stunning?

The new law would be an important step toward protecting our population. What will happen to it and the EPA in general under President Trump's reign is anyone's guess, but as I write this, it's not looking good. Not only is the fox in charge of the chicken coop, he is charging double for toxic eggs.

So more important than ever are the steps you take, dear reader, to take care of yourself and your family, without waiting for vested interests in Washington to have their sway.

Here is some well-researched advice from NRDC's reporter Alexandra Zissu about how to avoid the endocrine-disrupting chemicals that are the cause of many medical problems. I admit that some of her suggestions sound a bit extreme. But so does a diagnosis of breast cancer.

Turn up your nose at fragrances. Pretty smells can have ugly consequences, according to the research on a class of chemicals called phthalates, found in fragrances and countless consumer products.

Phthalates, even if you can't pronounce them, are endocrine disrupters. A few innocent sniffs and they're inside your body, mimicking hormones and creating havoc with your endocrine system, a network of hormones and glands that regulate everything you do.

So check labels, and when in doubt, buy fragrance-free.

Think twice about plastics. Many plastics are carriers of hormone-disrupting chemicals that harm your health, even at very low doses. BPA is one of the bad-boy plastics to avoid...but how? Clean up your act one step at a time: Replace plastic food containers with glass ones; never use plastic in the microwave; replace plastic baggies with reusable lunch bags and replace plastic cling wrap with beeswax-coated cloth. (I smile every time I cover half an apple with my reusable beeswax covers.)

Say no can do. This seems radical to me. No canned tuna? No baked beans? Zissu and the NRDC don't like cans of any sort, even those labeled "BPA-free." Don't use them, she writes. Choose fresh, frozen, or dried foods instead.

Rethink kid cosmetics. Zissu reports that kids are using personal care products more than ever, and just like the adult-kind, the kid-marketed cosmetics and lotions are packed with substances that get directly into the skin—the largest organ of the body—where they can do damage. Puberty, for instance, is coming on earlier than ever, and the complications aren't pretty. "Kids don't need cosmetics," Zissu reminds us. But the chemical industry always needs more customers, so that explains that.

Clean smarter. Don't get me started on household cleaners. Alexandra Zissu suggests you dispose of the harsh chemical and toxic kind immediately! And responsibly, of course.

For more than 40 years, we innocent zillions have been buying these big-bottle commercial cleaners and all their tainted cousins—oven cleaners, flame retardants— thinking they were harmless.

Oops.

The Toxic Substances Control Act of 1976 depended on the chemical industry of the U.S. to decide what's safe for consumers, aka "guinea pigs."

Let us agree they have not been doing a good job.

ENERGY EXPRESS-O! Better Living Through Chemistry?

"Not everything that is faced can be changed, but nothing can be changed until it is faced."
—James Baldwin

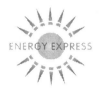

GOING DEEPER

If you can't trust the government to tell you what's safe and what's just aggressive marketing, who can you trust? That's the billion-dollar question. I'm not 100 percent sure what the answer is, but I will say, as a trained journalist from back in the day when journalists still had training, I trust the facts and findings at www.EWG.org, **a** website run by the Environmental Working Group.

What foods should you buy organic? Which lipsticks are the most toxic? When will the government get phthalates out of our food supply?

The EWG says it is a nonprofit, nonpartisan organization with more than 20 years experience in pursuit of their mission: "To empower people to live healthier lives in a healthier environment."

You'll find all sorts of useful information on the site, including the "Dirty Dozen," a list of the fruits and vegetables you absolutely must buy organic because the conventional kind are so laden with harmful pesticides.

Do you know what dangers lurk in your shampoo, your sunscreen, your storage containers? EWG does.

It's shocking, some of it—wait till you read the list of Dirty Dozen Endocrine Disruptors—but better to know what's really happening than wake up one day and wonder why your 7-year-old is developing breasts.

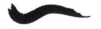

After my father died in 1999, I found a little piece of paper folded up and tucked away in his wallet. He'd scribbled down little truisms that inspired him to be the tender and trusted man he was. "Do your giving while you're living, then you'll be knowing where it's going," is one I treasure, right up there with Bob Dylan's famous line, "Those not busy being born are busy dying." What a great teaching. How could someone so brilliant be so rude, so petty, and not show up to accept his Nobel Prize for Literature in 2016? Dylan, not my Dad. What a dork. Everyone ages, but some people never grow up.

Age With Attitude.

Aging isn't just for old people. We all do it. And many of us, witnessing our sagging skin, muddled brain, the dreaded chin whiskers, just don't like it.

That's because most people don't see it the way Frank Lloyd Wright did.

"The longer I live," this world-famous architect believed, "the more beautiful life becomes."

More mysterious, too.

"The secret to staying young," Lucille Ball revealed, "is to live honestly, eat slowly, and lie about your age."

There must be 10 gazillion books on the subject of healthy aging. It's a multibillion-dollar industry that'll never die, even though every one of us will. That's why it's a compelling subject for all ages,

Instead of an overview, I'm going out on a limb to offer a point of view, my current nine rules—ideas? theories? self-delusions?—for healthy aging based on a lifetime of reading, writing, learning, exploring, and, oh, yeah, growing older.

Each rule could be a day's discussion or an eight-week online course. Forget that. The clock is ticking, space is limited, and I want to keep it simple. In fact, keeping it simple is the 10th rule.

The order is random, much like life. Number one is not more important than number nine, unless it is to you:

1. Expect success. Aging is not a disease. It's part of the natural flow of life. So embrace the positives about aging—wisdom and freedom are two biggies—and let go of the negative. People with positive perceptions of aging live seven years longer than people with negative perceptions. Not just longer, but happier, more meaningful lives. Seven years!

2. Exercise (mind and body). You can't hear this enough. To age gracefully, stay active. It's a must. Move it or it disappears. Walk, bike, swim, do yoga, whatever you like. Strength train, too. If you decide to run with only one of my so-called rules, make it this one.

3. Nourish your body. To age well, you have to eat well. That means real food, clean food, yummy food in amounts that don't make you sick or obese. The drama of dieting is over the day you give up processed foods, fake foods, sugary foods and let the healthiest part of you prepare and eat food that nourishes your body in a way that hot dogs and Pop-Tarts never will.

4. Accept what is. Strive to accept your life as it unfolds, without being angry or bitter, or feeling victimized. At the same time, fight hard to live the best, most-balanced life possible. Don't dwell in the past or obsess about the future. Live in the moment, and love the kind, compassionate person you are.

5. Rely on yourself. Self-care is the best care. Seek the finest medical care, but beware of overtreatment. Be smart about early detection and prevention, but avoid too much scrutiny. "What is a well person?" a doctor once asked his students. "A well person is a patient who hasn't been completely worked up."

6. Vent in healthy ways. Difficult things happen as you age. Sickness, pain, loss. You can't avoid the stress but you can, you must, learn to deal with it in healthy ways. Yoga, Qigong, meditation, exist for that purpose. Find your own practice, your own path, and you'll know you're on it when your anger turns to forgiveness, your jealousy to joy.

7. Take risks. If you want to feel vital, fully alive as you age, keep taking risks. Keep challenging yourself. Keep testing your limits. "Go out on a limb," Jimmy Carter said. "That's where the fruit is." When was the last time you went out on a limb?

8. Do unto others. The older and crankier you get, the more kindness and forgiveness have to come into play. Helping others adds more meaning and purpose to life. Love and be loved, and you will live longer, and die more gracefully.

9. Understand death and dying. All that is living comes to an end. It's not if, it's when. So delve into it with humor, curiosity, and spirit. Find a community that supports your choices and beliefs. And remember this: No one on a deathbed ever says, "I wish I'd spent more time at the office."

Now take the first letter for each rule—E-E-N-A-R-V-T-D-U—and play with the letters until you spell out a word that gets to the essence of healthy aging. Life's a great and mysterious game, and ultimately, just like aging, you have to unscramble it for yourself.

ENERGY EXPRESS-O! Everyone's an Expert

"The most important thing I can tell you about aging is this:
If you really feel that you want to have an off-the-shoulder
blouse and some big beads and thong sandals and
a dirndl skirt and a magnolia in your hair, do it.
Even if you're wrinkled."
—Maya Angelou

GOING DEEPER

I was asked to give a keynote speech about aging. Thinking it over, and over, and over again, I came up with these nine rules.

It wasn't easy. My first draft had 27. It was a 30-minute gig, so I did some heavy editing.

Now I'm happy I have them, and I'm asking you to do the same. Crafting your own rules, that is.

What have you learned about life that you want to pass on?

What matters most? What turns out not to matter at all?

It's hard to pare a lifetime of experience down to nine oversimplified guidelines, but do it anyway, even if you're young.

It's an exercise in figuring out what you know now. Start where you are.

Here's one thing I know: What matters most at the end of your life is who you love and who loves you.

I forgot to mention it in my nine.

You'll forget stuff, too, so write down your nine rules and keep them tucked away on a piece of paper, revising as you evolve, scribbling down new truths as they come to you.

You never know who'll find it one day, maybe in your wallet, and put it to very good use.

My dear sister—who reads my syndicated column regularly in the Gainesville Sun and is the kindest wisest sister a person could have—tells me that I write way too much about yoga. "Not everyone is interested," she reminds me. "You are, but other people aren't." She's right. I know that. But repetition brings rewards and the rewards of yoga are so many, I can't help but come back to it, time and time again, always finding some new little twist.

Protect Your Asanas.

Normally, my yoga class is an oasis of calm. We unroll our mats, gather our props, sit in a comfortable posture—unwinding, breathing, quieting our busy brains—and wait in silence for the teacher to begin.

Not this week. Holy Patanjali! A bomb had been dropped, and everyone was buzzing—not just in my yoga studio, but across the country:

"Did you see the piece in the Times?" "It was great!" "It was awful!" "Idiotic!" "Sensational!" "Can you believe that guy?"

That guy is William J. Broad, author of a highly inflammatory article in The New York Times magazine that turned the yoga community on its collective head.

Why? Because Broad focuses almost exclusively on the damage yoga can do if you're not careful—and sometimes, even if you are.

"A healthy women of 28 suffered a stroke while doing a yoga position known as the wheel," he writes, citing case after case of injuries, even though the sum total of documented yoga injuries is puny compared to running, basketball, and other athletic endeavors.

Broad isn't showing an interest in comparative studies. His article, adapted from his book "The Science of Yoga: The Risks and Rewards," warns people that "a number of commonly taught yoga poses are inherently risky."

Shoulder stand can "wreck havoc on the brain." Spinal twists can paralyze you. Bikram yoga can "raise the risk of overstretching, muscle damage and torn cartilage." And so on...

A story in The New York Times about the possibility of nuclear war with Iran gets 30 comments—on a good day. Broad's feature, called "All Bent Out of Shape: The Problem With Yoga," had 734 comments before you could say "Namaste."

Many of them were critical of Broad for his narrow view that ignored the benefits and philosophy of yoga in favor of the dangers. A few applauded him:

"I walked out of one of my first yoga classes with a double hernia," says Mike B. from Del Mar, California.

Amy from Montpelier, Vermont, was "appalled by his lack of research" and resented "the sensational and misleading photos" that showed the absolute wrong way to do popular yoga poses.

Charles from San Antonio called the article "deceptive and misleading and represents junk science...do not let this drivel discourage you from doing yoga."

"I started Bikram yoga when I was 64, about two years ago," writes injury-free Judy T. "My body has been transformed from being crippled and overweight to feeling energetic, strong and thin."

Annie from San Francisco thought Broad's article was "a great read."

Ditto from Clint, who prefers weight training to yoga: "Why put yourself in awkward, unnatural postures?" (Hello, Clint? Is a bench press a natural posture?)

And, finally, the gold star goes to Karan of Los Angeles who wrote the wisest reaction of all:

"It's not yoga that injures you, it's you that injures you. It's you not choosing the right teacher, it's you not being patient, it's you not listening to your body, it's you not taking responsibility, it's you passing your power to others."

My turn. I'm on a secret mission to get everyone to try yoga. Here's what I think:

All exercise involves risk. People can, and do, injure themselves doing all sorts of physical activities. Broad begins by saying he believed yoga could never harm you. That is foolish and naive. In truth, the greatest health risks come from doing no exercise at all.

Yoga in America has become a competitive sport. Yoga is an ancient, profound philosophy that connects body and mind with breath and leads to a calmer and healthier, happier life.

As Broad's article rightly points out, "If you do it with ego or obsession, you'll end up causing problems."

The injuries he dwells on can, for the most part, be prevented if you do yoga mindfully, with an experienced teacher, learning to pace yourself and never pushing into pain.

It's true there are many novice teachers—especially in gyms, with wall-to-wall mirrors—who are woefully underqualified and may push you into postures that your body can't handle.

It happens to everyone, until one day, you develop body awareness, move more slowly, trust your own boundaries, and intuit who can help you and who can hurt you.

Yoga isn't the enemy. Ignorance is. Do your asanas with *ahimsa,* Sanskrit for nonviolence: the first principal of yoga. Be kind to your body. Don't overstrain or overdo. Every body is different and finds strength, agility, and balance at its own relaxed pace.

When you accept your limitations, and celebrate what you *can* do, the joy of yoga is boundless.

ENERGY EXPRESS-O! Cloudless Thinking

"The way I see it, if you want the rainbow,
you gotta put up with the rain."
—Dolly Parton

GOING DEEPER

If you already do yoga, bravo! Please give yourself a pat on a previously unreachable part of your back.

If you don't do yoga, take a class. Not one—several to many. It can take a bit of time to begin to appreciate this wholly new way of relating to your body, to developing a felt sense of what it is about this ancient practice that is so restorative, so energizing, so transformational.

Read books; some terrific ones were written centuries ago, some yesterday.

Study with great teachers.

Subscribe to Yoga Journal, which has excellent articles on contemporary teachers and practice.

And move slowly, much more slowly than you think you should.

Above all, understand there is no "should" in yoga.

There is only yoga.

(I suspect my sister will say I've gone too far again. Deep bows to her.)

Some say the jury is out about the damage cellphone radiation is doing to our brains. That's because there is no real jury, not in the U.S., where cellphones have been judged as safe enough by the powers that be. And we are thankful that we have them, can't live without them, despite growing evidence that texting causes car crashes, and radiation overexposure is damaging, and young brains are being rewired in ways that put them at risk. Let's face (time) it: Unending distraction is the new normal and smartphones aren't going away. So what do we do? We become aware. We use the off button.

Outsmart Your Smartphone.

I know I'm sticking my neck out, but it's high time we take a deeper look at what lap-level technology is doing to our bodies as we spend hours and hours, day after day, year after year, looking down at our phones, our screens, and, now, our politicians.

Talk about shaping your destiny. The medical malady cutely called "Text Neck" is on the rise, as we conduct our lives on mobile devices—head forward, eyes lowered, shoulders slumped. It may sound harmless, but over time, this "downward-looking posture" has unintended and very expensive health care consequences. (This is more than a hunch.)

Neck and shoulder pain.

Chronic headaches and arthritis.

Pinched nerves and herniated discs.

Feelings of powerlessness and anxiety.

And that's not all.

"Think ADHD, immune issues, allergies, fatigue and hormone imbalances," Dr. Matt Thompson, a chiropractor based in Highlands Ranch, Colorado, emailed me recently. He is alarmed at what he's been seeing. And feeling.

"The advent and abundance of technology is skyrocketing 'forward head posture' and 'text neck' in the U.S. and worldwide," he said.

"Practically, this means any signal between brain and body, both function and feeling, can be affected."

Any signal between brain and body?! That can't be good. And it gets worse.

"Maintaining this forward head posture...stimulates the primitive brain while neglecting the higher brain," explained Dr. Thompson. "This creates an immature brain balance between the left and right hemispheres, which can lead to behavioral, social, and immune system issues."

By issues, he means problems.

Heavy is the head. The average adult head weighs between 10 and 12 pounds, depending on whether or not you were drinking the night before.

"For every inch the head goes forward beyond the shoulder, this is 10-15 extra pounds of stress and tension on the entire spine," says Dr. Thompson. He's talking about maybe 60 pounds hanging off your fragile neck, just so you can see the Pinterest posting of your friend's cat wearing a Cubs hat. "This can create pain, fatigue, soreness, headaches, vision and attention problems."

(I know I mentioned this earlier, but just in case you weren't paying attention...)

Text neck pressures your cervical spine. Text Neck, over time, can take the natural curve out of your neck, straighten your cervical spine, stretch the spinal cord and put pressure on your brainstem.

This is what sickness feels like, followed by pain, followed by millions of prescriptions for painkillers, which don't work well and tend to be addictive.

You're all connected. The slumped, looking-down-all-the-time posture isn't just bad for the body. It's also a big drag on your emotions, your spirit, your sense of power. That's the conclusion of many scientists, including social psychologist Amy Cuddy, associate professor at the Harvard Business School.

She's the best-selling author of "Presence" and presenter of a sensational 2012 TED Global talk seen by over 33 million viewers. I just hope you'll watch it with your eyes level at your standup desk.

As we know, the mind and body are connected. And so, Dr. Cuddy reports, when your body slumps, so do you, in subtle and debilitating ways. The Text Neck pose creates feelings of powerlessness and anxiety.

All this plus pain, fatigue, and stupidity.

OK, it's time for a serious heads-up.

Self-care is the best care. There are things you can do—besides quitting your job to bake bread in a Zen monastery—that can help you lower the boom on Text Neck and maybe prevent it.

—Read your screens at eye-level. Selfie sticks are useful, and so are adjustable device holders, easily found online. For desk work, get and USE a standup desk. For those times when you're out and about, just use your perfectly placed arms.

—Team up with savvy practitioners who specialize in the analysis and correction of spinal posture and speak the language of prevention.

—Take breaks, do stretches, train in a mind-body awareness practice such as yoga, Qigong, Alexander

Technique, Feldenkrais, or somatics so you can sense building tension before it explodes into chronic pain.

    —And this, dear readers: If you want to feel and act persuasively, and authentically, rise up from your screen slouch and follow Dr Cuddy's advice—strike the Power Pose: head up, eyes forward, shoulders wide, hands on hips, legs spread.

    Ain't no body gonna mess with you.

ENERGY EXPRESS-O!   Authenticity 'R' Us

"Let your body tell you you're powerful and deserving,
and you become more present, enthusiastic,
and authentically yourself."
—Amy Cuddy

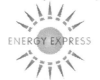

GOING DEEPER

    The Power Pose—also known as the Wonder Woman pose—involves standing tall, hands on hips, chest out. Don't be shy—it works just as well for men, boys, and girls, who often need it the most.

    And how exactly does it work? Amy Cuddy, among others, has proven that your body language impacts the level of testosterone and cortisol in your body. Wonder Woman raises your testosterone and lowers your cortisol.

Higher testosterone levels—in females and males—lead to greater confidence. Lower levels of cortisol make you feel less anxious and more able to deal with stress.

Wonder Woman positions you to be more assertive, more willing to take risks, more relaxed. It's the ideal thing to do every day—before school, an important meeting, a confrontation with a workplace creep.

You are how you stand. Strike this pose for two minutes a day for a couple of weeks, and zone in on how it makes you feel, inside, where only you can focus. Consider the following variation to make it even more effective.

While standing in the pose, close your eyes or gaze softly into the middle distance. Breathe in deeply for a count of four, hold for two, and then breathe out slowly to a count of five.

Wonder at how you feel: your sensations, your emotions. More open? More serene? Smile. It's the embodiment of All is Well.

"It's not that I'm afraid to die—I just don't want to be there when it happens." I laugh whenever I hear Woody Allen's confession, but my thinking has evolved. I was there when my mother died. And I was there when my father died. And I want to be there when I die. Arranging that in a society hell-bent on turning dying into a problem to be solved isn't easy, but it's more and more possible. If you've ever worked with hospice, you know what a blessing palliative care is—one of the kindest things to happen to health care over the last 40 years. I'm happy to report the country's interest in death and dying is more alive than ever.

Start the Conversation.

Have you had the Conversation?

Probably not. Most people don't, until it's too late.

However, more people are. It feels good, once you get started. But getting started can be tricky.

I began the Conversation in the kitchen of my niece's house a while back. A 90-year-old elder we both knew had died and I found myself saying that the way Dorris died—in her bed, surrounded by loving family and friends, no fear, no pain, touched and held until the end—was a blessing, not only in her life, but in mine, too. It inspired me to cue the harps and face the music when it comes to thinking about, and planning for, my own final breath.

And that's what the Conversation is—an honest and open discussion with your loved ones about what you do and do not want when it comes to end-of-life care.

The Conversation isn't written in stone. It will evolve as you do: home care or hospital? the Beatles or Bach?

candles or cannabis or both? The end-of-life Conversation is personal, and private, but it needs to happen while you're healthy, because when the time comes to really spell out the details, you might be too late.

"It's always too soon until it's too late," writes Ellen Goodman, the Pulitzer Prize-winning journalist who co-founded The Conversation Project, a "public engagement campaign with a goal that is both simple and transformative: to have every person's end-of-life wishes expressed and reported."

What a heavenly idea!

"It's not surprising that we postpone and postpone these conversations. Talking about dying is hard," Goodman says. "When I opened the subject with my own daughter Katie, her first response was 'Can't we just have lunch?'" Goodman isn't joking when she writes and speaks about the heart-wrenching experience of her mother's death and the enormous gap between what people say they want at the end of life, and what actually happens.

Here are some eye-opening statistics from The Conservation Project, in collaboration with the Institute for HealthCare Improvement:

—70 percent of people say they prefer to die at home...but in fact, 70 percent of people die in a hospital, nursing home or long-term care facility.

—80 percent of people say if seriously ill they would want to talk to their doctor about end-of-life care...but in fact, only 7 percent report having had end-of-life conversations with their doctor.

—90 percent of Americans know they should have a conversation about what they want at the end of life...yet only 30 percent have done so.

If so many people want to have the Conversation, why isn't it happening?

One reason, according to The Conversation Project's recent survey, is that people simply don't know how to get it going.

Imagine a family gathering. It's Thanksgiving, the perfect time to be grateful for the life you have and the end-of-life care you want. But how do you pause the football game and begin? What do you say?

And that's where the Conversation Project's end-of-life starter kit comes into play. It's a free download from their website, a well-written, step-by-step guide that gives you tools, medical directives, resources, and more than a few questions to get the Conversation going.

Here, for instance, are some questions a son or daughter might ask an aging parent before he or she gets a diagnosis, before they end up in intensive care:

"When you think about the last phase of your life, what's most important to you?"

"When would it be OK to shift from a focus on curative care to a focus on comfort care?"

"On a scale of one to five, with one being 'I want to live as long as possible, no matter what' and five being 'Quality of life is more important to me than quantity,' where do you stand? "

"We want you to be the expert on your wishes and those of your loved ones," the Conversation Project makes clear. "Not the doctors or nurses. Not the end-of-life experts. You."

The starter kit gets you talking, and just as crucially, it gets you listening.

Listen to what your spouse wants, your brother, your best friend. Listen without judging. Just listen. And listen to your own answers when you're having the Conversation. The more you talk through the details of your own desires, the better you'll feel.

That's been my experience, beginning in my niece's kitchen that day, and I'd bet my life it'll be true for you.

"This isn't about dying," the experts say about having the Conversation. "It's about figuring out how you want to live till the very end."

ENERGY EXPRESS-O! You Be the Decider

"In being with dying, we arrive at a natural crucible of what it means to love and be loved. And we can ask ourselves this: Knowing that death is inevitable, what is most precious today?"
—Joan Halifax

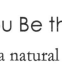

GOING DEEPER

Dr. Atul Gawande—a surgeon and professor at Harvard Medical School—has written a magnificent book about death and dying called "Being Mortal." It's a best-seller with a cult following, an acknowledgement that doctors in America are taught to see death as a failure. It reminds you, the reader, to take end-of-life matters into your own hands, your own heart, if you want to exit with grace and gratitude.

"You don't have to spend much time with the elderly or those with terminal illness to see how often medicine fails the people it is supposed to help," Gawande writes. "The waning days of our lives are given over to treatments that addle our brains and sap our bodies for a sliver's chance of benefit."

As soon as I finished reading "Being Mortal," I started it again. And then I bought a copy for everyone in my family, and then all my friends, and then I told strangers on airplanes to read it, and now...you. It's that good.

Another brilliant book to help you go deeper into dying was written by my friend Roshi Joan Halifax, founder of the Upaya Institute and Zen Center. It's called "Being With Dying: Cultivating Compassion and Fearlessness in the Presence of Death," a classic published in 2009 and now the foundation of a training program taught in hundreds of medical and educational institutions around the world.

We all want a "good death," but the truth is we're going to get the death we get, Roshi Joan teaches.

So how do we make the most of that, without judging, without suffering to extremes, with clarity and acceptance and love?

Her wise guidance on this most delicate and profound subject sheds light and perspective on this greatest of mysteries, our final adventure.

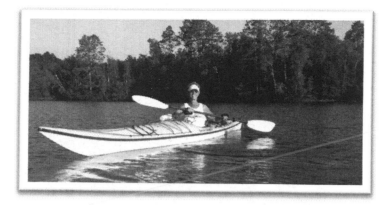

Acknowledgements

Let me close first with deep bows to the entire team at Creators Publishing—led by Jack Newcombe, Rick Newcombe, and my diligent in-house book editor with the lightest touch, Simone Slykhous. They inspired and encouraged me to write this book. And Simone took my running puns in stride.

Also—luckily this isn't an awards show with music rising to rush my thanks—I want to express boundless gratitude to my unconditionally loving parents, my sister, my entire, ever expanding family, every dear friend, every teacher, every interview, every training, every book I've read and yoga class I've taken, and yes, thank you to the intrepid husband I rode bicycles in France with and was married to for 35 years.

All of them and all of it enabled me to discover, cherish and not shy from the path to my own well-being.

And who more than Barbara? My adored editor-in-chief, who introduced me to the bliss of eating crispy fries, riding bikes that are really our ponies, and trusting the sea even when you can't see to the bottom. We married in 2014, on the spring equinox.

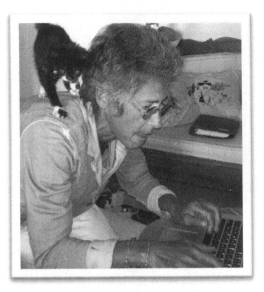

About the Author

Marilynn Preston—journalist, healthy lifestyle expert, Emmy Award-winning TV producer—is the author of "Energy Express," America's longest-running syndicated fitness column.

In her engaging, opinionated style, Marilynn explores what it means to live a healthy, happy lifestyle. From eating clean to going green, she links body and mind to politics and culture, and always encourages readers to start where they are.

Marilynn is an ACE-certified fitness trainer and certified Wellcoach, and she has written two other books, "Dear Dr. Jock: The People's Guide to Sports and Fitness" and "Work Well, Be Well." She created, exec produced and co-wrote the nationally syndicated "Energy Express" TV series about sports, fitness, and adventure for kids and families. For this work, she won two Emmys and a Women's Sports Foundation award for outstanding programming.

Marilynn is also the founding chair of a life-changing nonprofit called Girls in the Game. More than 20 years later, she still works as a relentless board member, helping girls get the healthy lifestyle training they need to become strong, confident, powerful women. Please visit www.girlsinthegame.org to meet the girls, hear their remarkable stories, and make a donation. (Told you she was relentless.)

When Marilynn isn't writing, her healthy lifestyle routine includes yoga, race walking, strength training, kayaking, golf, cycling, wine tasting and as much adventure travel as she can fit in. She's circumambulated Mt. Kailash in Tibet, climbed Mt. Olympus in Greece, bicycled in France and Italy, golfed in Bhutan, and scuba dived in the YMCA pool in Chicago.

Her next big adventure is getting people to read All is Well to create their healthiest, happiest lives.

All Is Well

The Art {and Science} of Personal Well-Being
is also available as an e-book for Kindle,
Amazon Fire, iPad, Nook, and Android e-readers.
Visit creatorspublishing.com to learn more.

o o o

CREATORS PUBLISHING

737 3rd St.
Hermosa Beach, CA
310-337-7003

o o o

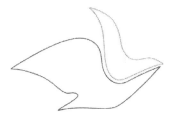

Made in the USA
Lexington, KY
20 July 2017